A PLUME BOOK

HEALTHY CHILD HEALTHY WORLD

CHRISTOPHER GAVIGAN is chief executive officer of Healthy Child Healthy World. For more than a decade he has dedicated himself to improving the lives of children and families. He holds degrees in environmental science and geography from the University of California, Santa Barbara, and has extensive graduate training in child psychology and education. He has worked as a children and family specialist and is the founder of Pinnacle Expeditions, an outdoor leadership program for teenagers.

Since joining Healthy Child Healthy World, Gavigan has launched public awareness campaigns and programs that have educated millions about daily choices and action that affect our children's health and our planet's future.

Healthy Child Healthy World

CREATING A CLEANER, GREENER, SAFER HOME

FOREWORD BY MERYL STREEP

Christopher Gavigan

CEO, HEALTHY CHILD HEALTHY WORLD

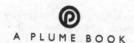

A PLUME BOOK

PLUME
Published by the Penguin Group
Penguin Group (USA) Inc., 375 Hudson Street, New York, New York 10014, U.S.A. • Penguin Group (Canada), 90 Eglinton Avenue East, Suite 700, Toronto, Ontario, Canada M4P 2Y3 (a division of Pearson Penguin Canada Inc.) • Penguin Books Ltd., 80 Strand, London WC2R 0RL, England • Penguin Ireland, 25 St. Stephen's Green, Dublin 2, Ireland (a division of Penguin Books Ltd.) • Penguin Group (Australia), 250 Camberwell Road, Camberwell, Victoria 3124, Australia (a division of Pearson Australia Group Pty. Ltd.) • Penguin Books India Pvt. Ltd., 11 Community Centre, Panchsheel Park, New Delhi – 110 017, India • Penguin Group (NZ), 67 Apollo Drive, Rosedale, North Shore 0632, New Zealand (a division of Pearson New Zealand Ltd.) • Penguin Books (South Africa) (Pty.) Ltd., 24 Sturdee Avenue, Rosebank, Johannesburg 2196, South Africa

Penguin Books Ltd., Registered Offices: 80 Strand, London WC2R 0RL, England

Published by Plume, a member of Penguin Group (USA) Inc. Previously published in a Dutton edition.

First Plume Printing, April 2009
10   9   8   7   6   5   4   3

Permissions appear on page 302 and constitute an extension of the copyright page.

The Library of Congress has catalogued the Dutton edition as follows:

Gavigan, Christopher.
Healthy child, healthy world: creating a cleaner, greener, safer home / foreword by Meryl Streep; by Christopher Gavigan.
p. cm.
Includes bibliographical references and index.
ISBN 978-0-525-95047-9 (hc.)
ISBN 978-0-452-29019-8 (pbk.)
1. Home economics—Handbooks, manuals, etc.
2. Children—Health and hygiene.   3. Housing and health—Popular works.   4. Ecological houses—Health aspects.   5. Sustainable living—Handbooks, manuals, etc.   6. Natural products.   I. Title.
TX145.G284   2008
640—dc22   2007050535

Printed in the United States of America
Original hardcover design by Chris Welch

For my son,
Luke Hudson Gavigan,
and the children of today and tomorrow:

May the nourishment of the earth be yours,
may the clarity of light be yours,
may the fluency of the ocean be yours,
may the protection of the ancestors be yours.

—JOHN O'DONOHUE, *Anam Cara*

CONTENTS

There's a saying in Bangladesh about the theater: To be a good actor, you should know the words and movements and execute them perfectly; to be a great actor, you should know the words and movements and execute them perfectly, and also be able to invest them with great meaning; but to be a master actor, you should know the words and movements and execute them perfectly, invest them with great meaning, and be a farmer.

I am an actress, not a farmer. But as a mother, I've had my hands in the dirt and my eyes on the sky the whole time. I'm a caretaker and a cultivator of a sort, and I think the wisdom in the adage above applies not just to acting but to parenting, as well.

As a parent, you always try to do the right thing. You teach your kids not only how to take care of themselves, but to look for meaning in what they do, and to contribute to society. You also understand that the "right" environment in which to raise healthy children is a healthy environment—a place where the earth that feeds them (and us), the air they breathe, and the water they drink and bathe in are not poisoned. You don't have to be a farmer to know this.

In 1989, when my children were three, six, and ten years old, I read a report from the Natural Resources Defense Council entitled *Intolerable*

Risk. It outlined the risks posed to infants and children by pesticide residues on fruits and vegetables. One chemical dominated the statistics—Alar, a substance that was sprayed on apples to regulate growth and enhance color, and had been under review by the Environmental Protection Agency for three years previous. The American Academy of Pediatrics had already recommended that it be banned. Alar was a systemic additive—meaning it could not be washed off—and it had strong cancer-causing properties so it presented an accumulating threat to growing bodies over the long term. Babies, children, and pregnant women were especially at risk. The faster metabolism of developing babies, and, pound for pound, their greater relative intake of these residues were troubling. Together with other exposures to toxic chemicals in the physical environment, this threat to children's health needed to be communicated broadly.

I gathered some of my Connecticut neighbors and we formed a group called Mothers and Others to inform other parents about the findings of this report. We began in our town, alerting and educating families, then got the word out to others—grocery stores, restaurants, relatives, and friends. We wanted to change the way toxic chemicals were regulated, we wanted better access to foods that were not "treated," and we wanted to let parents know that even a healthy diet of fruits and vegetables (among other things) might contain certain substances that could cross the placenta and affect their unborn children. That once the child was born these toxic chemicals would enter their bodies via breast milk. That, once weaned, those little bodies would take in foods that might contain substances that could prove problematic to their health, and to their mental and reproductive capacity later in their lives.

Because of my media access, I was able to get the word out via speeches, television appearances, and testimony before Congress. Our group, with the support and guidance of numerous other committed and informed individuals and groups, successfully campaigned against the use of the chemical Alar. Not only that, but broader benefits came out of our campaign:

- In 1993, after a five-year study brought into being by the Alar controversy, the National Academy of Sciences confirmed children's unique and heightened vulnerabilities in its report *Pesticides in the Diet of Infants and Children.*
- Previous to this, allowable levels for pesticide residue in the body were based on data from full-grown men. After this report, the tolerances were changed to reflect children's special vulnerabilities, and President Clinton signed new regulations into law.

Mothers and Others expanded its scope and began tackling other environmental dangers. Again, we proceeded on the logic that if some substance or activity has a damaging effect on adults, then it's almost certainly worse for kids. We learned from people like Dr. Philip Landrigan, professor of pediatrics and director of the Center for Children's Health and the Environment at the Mount Sinai School of Medicine, who examined the health hazards of persistent organic pollutants, heavy metals, and air pollutants on children. Childhood cancer is up about 25 percent in the last generation. American children are harmed by air pollution, which reduces their respiratory capacity, rendering them more vulnerable to colds and ear infections. In recent years, the incidence of asthma has surged; more than six million children now suffer from it. One in every thirty-three babies born in the United States enters the world with a birth defect. One in six children deals with at least one developmental disorder. Between 3 and 5 percent have Attention Deficit Hyperactivity Disorder. While these troubling increases can't wholly be attributed to environmental poisons, there are measures we all can take to reduce risk. But we need a reliable guide to help us identify those risks—how to avoid them and what to do to offset their potential impact. This book can be that guide.

Healthy Child Healthy World helps mothers and fathers connect the dots, to understand cause and effect. It came into existence not just to inform the public but to energize it. As a nonprofit organization, Healthy Child's mission is "prevention through education," according to cofounder Nancy Chuda, whose daughter Colette's death at age five, of a nongenetic form of cancer called Wilms' tumor, served as catalyst for the organization's creation.

I met Nancy in the late 1980s when, as a reporter for the TV program *The Home Show*, she covered some of Mothers and Others' campaign against pesticides. Later, when her daughter got sick, the tragedy spurred Nancy and her husband, Jim, to found Healthy Child Healthy World (formerly Children's Health Environmental Coalition). She, Jim, and the Healthy Child team were dedicated, as she said, "to preventing the cause so that we don't have children getting so sick" in the first place. "Parents can learn simple things to do in their homes, backyards, schools, and communities to make a really big difference, a difference that could save a life."

Healthy Child Healthy World helps parents focus on what we can do right now as *individuals*. So much that's out there now is about what you should *not* do; Healthy Child tries to emphasize the healthful solutions, the positive, easy-to-follow steps you can take for your family, your home, yourself. Of course, the steps we take at home have larger ramifications, because the choices we make every day at the grocery store and the hardware store count. With each purchase we make (and don't make), we're all voting for a more healthful (or safer) environment. It's an extremely effective way we have of demanding safer, better products and practices.

Why is the truth like organic food? Because it's a little harder to find, and a little more expensive than the alternative, but as demand for it grows, the price you have to pay for it comes down . . .

With a book like this, it's getting easier to find.

—Meryl Streep

Healthy Child
Healthy World

Your (Kids') Health Is Your Wealth

If a disease is made by human beings, we can prevent it.
—Dr. Philip Landrigan, director, Center for Children's Health
and the Environment, Mount Sinai School of Medicine,
Healthy Child Healthy World board member

W hen I first described this book to my mother, she said, "Oh, it's about how much you love your children." I can't put it better.

With parenthood comes a most spectacular wake-up call. This beautiful, mysterious, squirmy creature emerges—and so does our primal need to protect that miracle: to keep him healthy; to help her learn and engage with the world; to make him feel comforted and secure; to get her to belly-laugh. So you do what any thoughtful, motivated, loving—okay, and maybe slightly obsessive—parent does. You crawl across the floor, clutching plug covers, sticking them in every outlet. You pore over books about sleep schedules. You hang dangling toys meant to stimulate. The vigilance never ends: From rules about street and helmet safety to negotiations over eating veggies before ice cream, you're prepared. You're a parent. You will let no harm come to this child.

I'm a parent—a new parent, no less. I heard the wake-up call. And as CEO of Healthy Child Healthy World, I know the call has a double alarm. Yet many parents, even those environmentally minded among us who recycle, turn off unneeded lights, and conserve water, are only just grasping a second aspect so crucial to their children's well-being: protection from harmful chemicals and contaminants in the world around them. Here at

Healthy Child, we're fortunate to have access to a vast store of information—compiled and reviewed by some of the world's leading environmental scientists, pediatricians, and children's health advocates—that can help us all. And we *do* need help: with the air children breathe, the food they eat, the toys they play with, the materials and fabrics they sit and lie on, the grass they run through. More than eighty thousand synthetic chemicals are registered for use today, and several thousand are found in our everyday environments. While many of these chemicals are beneficial, far too few of them have been tested for toxicity. We don't know the extent of the risks they pose or how they interact, but we do know there are risks—and more are being uncovered each day. Unwittingly, we are all exposed to different recipes, soups of countless chemicals—many at a time, all the time.

42 billion number of pounds of chemicals the United States produces or imports each day. That's 140 pounds per person—every day. (National Pollution Prevention and Toxics Advisory Committee, 2005)

Your child may never stick his finger in an electrical outlet—especially the one behind the couch you strained your neck to get to—but you're doing what you can to take precautions by covering it. And "precaution" is the operative term here. How long should we wait for more definitive studies to come along showing harmful relationships between certain chemicals and health? Next year? Ten years from now? It took decades of research to show conclusively that cigarette smoking causes cancer and heart disease, yet it was highly suspected for years. In environmental science, we frequently invoke the "precautionary principle"—a fancy way of saying "better safe than sorry." Healthy Child maintains that we must be cautious right now about protecting our children from substances that may well prove harmful sometime down the road.

An electrical outlet is a physical reality. You can see it, touch it; you understand what it does and its potential to harm, because you can actually witness it. But chemicals are often not like that. They're not tangible or detectable in that way. Often they're invisible. Sometimes they give off a telltale smell, sometimes not. It's hard to appreciate fully that some microscopic, nebulous molecules can harm your child, especially when your rosy-cheeked tot is scampering across the floor, an energetic bubble of health. Inevitably you start to wonder how much attention you really need to pay to certain environmental factors. "Do I really need to be *that* cautious?" you ask yourself. "Since I'm healthy, won't my children be, too?"

Child development is a precise, delicate process. Kids between one and five eat three to four times more food per pound of body weight than the average adult; by the same measure, the air intake of a resting infant is twice that of an adult. Children absorb more nutrients and, consequently, more toxins than we do. Because their metabolic systems are still developing, their ability to detoxify and excrete harmful chemicals differs from that of adults, often leaving them more vulnerable to substances we all encounter. What's more, children and babies are more likely than adults to come in contact with these contaminants in the first place, since they spend more time on or close to the ground, indoors and out. And infants explore by putting everything into their mouths.

Just like the absorption of good nutrients, initial exposure to bad chemicals starts early, at conception (or even *before*): Some chemicals in a pregnant woman's body can cross the placenta and affect her growing baby during critical stages of development. Indeed, the harm posed by some chemicals is much greater during pregnancy than at any point in the human lifespan. With adult-scale chemical quantities transported to a tiny fetus, our offspring end up shouldering a far larger share of today's increasing chemical legacy, or "body burden," than adults do. Meanwhile, childhood diseases, from asthma to cancer, are on the rise. While the causes of these chronic conditions are complex, the role environmental exposures play in these illnesses has become increasingly apparent.

Here, I want to introduce a precautionary principle of my own, something I've deduced from countless stories we hear at Healthy Child: *Don't get overwhelmed.* When potential harm lurks, that urge to protect can send any parent into a frenzy. Instead, take a deep breath and know that, as with the plug covers, you have more control over the situation than you think, and it's never too late to start. Every generation has had its pitfalls. The 1950s—those happy, supposedly carefree days of Ozzie and Harriet—gave us houses filled with cigarette smoke and lead paint, and pesticide trucks that blanketed neighborhoods as children skipped down the streets, dancing in the spray. Today, in the twenty-first century, we're lucky. Over the past couple of decades, scientists, government, and industry (yes, many of them *are* good guys) have brought us sound research. We also have an ever-growing array of nontoxic products to keep our children safe. With information, we tremendously improve the odds of staying healthy.

And that's what this book offers: information and easy steps to help you understand the benefits of following some eminently doable steps— steps you can take at your pace, in your home, to keep your children safe. For almost two decades, Healthy Child has collected, distilled, and translated important scientific information related to our children's physical well-being. In this book, we've added for guidance the voices of many world-class experts in environmental health, as well as the practical experiences of parents. I have to admit that, with this information, I feel I can protect my baby son much better.

That said, it's important to comprehend the world our children live in. Here are some facts that should motivate us to action:

- **Cancer.** The incidence of childhood cancers jumped almost 27 percent between 1975 and 2002. While survival rates have skyrocketed, the cures come at a cost. Treatments kill cancer cells, but they damage healthy cells as well, causing complications from heart problems and liver failure to infertility. Survivors of childhood cancer have a mortality rate more than ten times higher than the general population's due to the long-term effects of treatment. The American Cancer Society estimates that 75 percent of cancer is due to environmental factors: Exposure to pesticides, hazardous air pollutants, and formaldehyde increase the risk of childhood cancers, while other exposures can raise a child's risk for adult onset cancers. But there is still much we need to learn about this connection.

- **Asthma.** According to the U.S. Centers for Disease Control and Prevention, in 2005, 6.5 million children under age eighteen had asthma, an increase of more than 200 percent since 1980. About one in eleven school-aged children suffers from asthma, and the rate is rising more rapidly in *preschool*-aged children than in any other age group. Indoor air quality is a big culprit. In addition to dust mites, mold, pet dander, and secondhand smoke, air contaminants that may contribute to asthma include certain insecticides and chemicals in plastic, especially formaldehyde.

- **Allergies.** Allergies have become widespread over the past several decades. Allergic dermatitis (itchy rash) is one of the most common skin conditions in children younger than eleven, and the percentage of children diagnosed with it increased more than 300 percent from the 1960s to the 1990s. Hay fever (allergic rhinitis) is believed to affect up to 40 percent of children; each day, approximately ten thousand American children miss school because of hay fever, for a total of 2 million lost school days a year. And roughly 6 percent of children suffer from food allergies, according to the CDC.

- **Autism and ADHD.** Diagnoses for autism and Attention Deficit Hyperactivity Disorder have jumped almost 400 percent in the last twenty years, according to a study published in the *American Journal of Psychiatry*. This increase is too high to attribute simply to improved recognition and diagnosis. Also, while causes of these disorders are complex, many chemicals, including lead, mercury, PCBs, alcohol, and other solvents are known to interfere with brain development.

- **Mental development and retardation.** The Environmental Protection Agency (EPA) estimates that at least 200,000 children born each year in the United States suffer mild to moderate loss of IQ points because of methylmercury exposure during fetal development; there has also been strong evidence for IQ loss from PCBs. The main source for both is mom's fish consumption during pregnancy. Meantime, many other inadequately tested industrial chemicals have the potential to disrupt childhood brain development.

- **Hormone disruption.** Endocrine disruptors—often found in plastics and cosmetics—mimic or block hormones, disrupting normal function, and have been shown to cause birth defects in laboratory animals. While evidence of human harm is unclear, some types of birth defects appear to be increasing, and more research is urgently needed.

- **Obesity.** Poor diet and lack of exercise have contributed to an epidemic of childhood obesity. One in six American children between the ages of six and nineteen are considered overweight, according to the U.S. surgeon general. Type 2 diabetes, once known as adult-onset diabetes, is increasing among children: One in three children born in the year 2000 will develop diabetes; for an African-American or Latino baby, the ratio is closer to one in two. And the cause is not just poor diet: Studies have shown that chemicals, like Bisphenol A (BPA), found in some plastics—such as water bottles—may interfere with normal hormone function, making obesity more likely.

🍃 Expert Opinion 🍃
The Best Prevention
By Dr. Harvey Karp, pediatrician, author/creator of the book/DVD
The Happiest Toddler on the Block, and
Healthy Child Healthy World board member

Caring for a baby is the sweetest, most beautiful experience a person can have. But, having been a pediatrician for thirty years, I know that parenting is also a big challenge. Even as we lovingly focus on feeding and soothing our infants, we have to start thinking about the next big job—keeping them healthy and safe. A safe home not only protects babies from dangers we can see, like stairs and sharp corners, but also from dangers we can't, like pesticides and other unhealthy chemicals.

As the months go by, you'll be amazed at how many times you'll say to your child, "Be careful!" Caution is also the sacred rule taught to doctors on the first day of training: *Primum non nocere. Above all, do no harm.* For environmental scientists working to protect kids, this essential call to "be careful" is dubbed the "precautionary principle" (something you'll hear emphasized throughout this book).

Every year, we learn that things once thought to be harmless can have serious, even disastrous consequences. No one ever dreamed that asbestos sprayed on ceilings could cause fatal lung disease. Or that hairspray could damage the ozone layer and contribute to a worldwide epidemic of skin cancer. Yet both occurred.

John Muir, the great American naturalist, said that if you reach out and tug on a tiny piece of nature, you'll discover that everything is connected to everything else. And because of this great connection, we often blunder into doing harm. . . . "Oops, we didn't know the chemical we were using caused cancer!" . . . "Oops, we're sorry we polluted your river for the next one hundred years!" Unintended consequences like these are especially worrisome for children because their early life experiences and exposures can affect whether or not they will grow up to have healthy and happy lives.

Statistics show that the average American is living longer—and that's great—but many of us don't share in this blessing. As you will learn in this book, several serious childhood illnesses and ailments, from cancer to asthma to birth defects to autism, are on the rise.

Are some of these growing health threats to our children triggered by environmental exposures? We don't know for sure, but for many years worrisome evidence of an association between chemical exposures and these health problems has been mounting. The evidence is solid and should compel us to take action, yet woefully little is being done. Why is there such inaction? In large part it's because the government lets products be sold as long as they haven't been *proven* to cause harm. But unlike you and me, chemicals should never be considered innocent until proven guilty; in fact, we must consider them *guilty* until proven *innocent*! We must demand that the industry prove a substance safe before it is allowed to be sold to millions.

Unfortunately, we do not have that level of protection today. However, some hope is on the horizon. A new federal program may bring us closer to the protection we deserve: The National Children's Study. This seminal investigation will study how industrial chemicals affect our kids' health. The project will measure chemicals in the blood of one hundred thousand babies and then follow the health of these children for twenty years, looking for any links between chemicals and illness. It is expected that within just the first years of this work, some of today's pressing questions, such as, "Is there a chemical link to autism?" will begin to find answers.

In the meantime, we have lots of reasons for being optimistic. Over just the past twenty years, we've removed tons of lead from paint and gasoline, started huge recycling programs, encouraged millions to stop smoking, banned asbestos, made organic food more widely available, designed cars that go fifty miles on a gallon of gas, and learned to prevent skin cancer with sunscreen and avoidance.

We've changed the world before. For the sake of our kids, it's time to do it again. In this book you'll find lots of great ways to boost health, shrink risks, and stack the deck in your child's favor.

So, congratulations! You're now an official member of the huge and growing community of parents across our great country, and our great world, who have made a commitment to give their children a living legacy of sparkling good health and a sparkling healthy planet. Now, let's all roll up our sleeves and go to work!

Minor Changes, Major Payoff

Reading through all these statistics about childhood illnesses can make your head hurt—some may find it downright terrifying. But here's the thing: Small, simple changes can yield big payoffs. And I see it all the time.

Before I joined Healthy Child, I did my academic work in environmental sciences, education, and child psychology, and worked in the Los Angeles area with families of children with special needs—kids struggling with breathing difficulties, learning delays, and developmental problems. Even though I was relatively unseasoned in the field, right away I saw how making small changes to the home environment really can improve the health of a family, and how truly doable these solutions are.

In one instance, I worked with a boy suffering from asthma and a variety of behavioral problems who was greatly helped—he started to breathe easier, grew calmer, and became more focused at school—when the overbearing artificially fragranced candles and deodorizers throughout his home were removed. (His mother kept vanilla-scented products in nearly every room—vanilla plug-in deodorizers, vanilla candles, vanilla fabric sprays, vanilla-scented potpourri sitting in dishes on tables.) Such artificial fragrances tend to contain chemicals that can irritate lungs, and perhaps even contribute to chronic disease down the line. In another situation, a girl I worked with had incredibly sensitive skin—full-body rashes, persistent itching, infections, acne. She'd been tested for all kinds of allergies but none were found. So her chemical exposure was reduced: Her parents purged their home of harsh, synthetic cleaners and phosphate-loaded laundry detergent. Her conventional body creams, which contained skin-irritating chemicals, gave way to organic alternatives. Her new synthetic, polyurethane-filled bed, loaded with flame retardants that could be irritating in the short run (and whose unhealthy effects just aren't fully known), was replaced with a comfortable, organic cotton mattress. Within three months her skin cleared up remarkably.

Simply removing a few chemicals won't solve everything that ails us. But here at Healthy Child, we hear about many, many sick children who recover from illness after their parents make some easy modifications in the home. I've seen firsthand how profoundly the environment affects children—afflicting them with asthma, behavior problems, chronic runny noses, and sore throats. But I've also seen just as vividly how replacing what's damaging in the environment can mean a huge, often life-altering benefit. The precautionary principle *can* work.

No One Can Do Everything.
Everyone Can Do Something.

What, then, are the most important, practical, effective things we can do for our children? Where do we start? What are the shortcuts? Each of the ten chapters that follow deals with a different aspect of your home environment—from cleaning products and food to toys, gardening, and home improvement—and breaks it down into ten totally doable steps. I encourage you to do as much or as little as you want. Some parents may decide to convert to organic, pesticide-free food first, and others might want to install a whole-house water filter or cut back on the plastics in the house. Do what feels comfortable. Taking even one step is a great stride. No one can do everything, but everyone can do something.

Our facts, as I mentioned, have been vetted by scientific and medical experts. (Should you want to know more about the sources used, go to our Web site, healthychild.org/booknotes.) Just as important, this book includes the voices of contributing parents, both well known and unfamiliar, who feel the way you do, who are going through what you are, who share successes to inspire and failures to learn from. Many people are acting on their kids' behalf, using safer products and trying their best. Now you can, too. To make this process easier, the Healthy Resources section at the back of the book lists recommended brands, services, Web sites, and helpful organizations to get you started. And if you want a more hard-core understanding of any of the terms in this book, log on to healthychild.org/glossary.

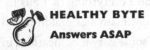 **HEALTHY BYTE**
Answers ASAP

At our award-winning Web site, healthychild.org, find daily tips and news from health experts, along with many useful features: blog, videos, community discussion forums, hundreds of easy-to-understand articles, podcasts, and up-to-date information on green, nontoxic products and services.

Parentblog
Generation Green
By Amy Brenneman, actress, Healthy Child Healthy World advisory board member

My dad has been an environmental lawyer and activist since the sixties. Growing up, we recycled, my mother dried the clothes outside (even in the dead of winter in New England), and we kept the house at 68 degrees. That's what's odd to me now—in the early and mid-seventies there was such an environmental movement happening. We would be competitive about our parents' fuel-efficient cars, and in seventh-grade shop class I silk-screened a T-shirt that said "Ecology for America." Then what happened—the eighties? We couldn't follow through? It's strange to see some of these things that emerged thirty years ago now presented as new.

I became involved with Healthy Child Healthy World because of my dad's work (he's part of something called Environment and Human Health out of Yale University) and because, of course, I became a mom myself. We started cleaning with Method products, we stopped chemical pest and weed control, we started eating more organic foods. The first day our pest guy came and used organic methods was so moving to me. I expected to have to clear out of my office for the requisite four hours, but he, maskless, said no. That wasn't necessary since no harsh chemicals were being used. A lightbulb went on. Oh, my god, I said. "This is so much better for you guys, too!" He beamed. Of course: Imagine being around that stuff all day?

I drive a Prius, often with two kids in back. I laugh, thinking that everyone feels like they need a tank out here in L.A. to cart around two small people. We also recently installed a huge water filter so we can actually drink our water, and I've been buying refillable metal bottles to get rid of the hundreds of plastic bottles that used to litter our house.

But we're not perfect. I tried my two-year-old on gDiapers and he looked at me like, no way. Not that they're not great; I just think now is not the time to start the guy on a new kind of diaper, when he's just about to give up diapers for good. It's hard to rid the house of plastics—we still have our Tupperware. And our eating could be better. Not being much of a cook, I'm more dependent on prepared foods than I'd like to be.

I think the biggest emotional struggle is not getting overwhelmed. Healthy Child sponsored a talk with Dr. Theo Colborn, who authored *Our Stolen Future*, which is about things like endocrine disrupters causing male fish in Lake Erie to grow ovaries—that kind of thing—and tying it into the alarming rates of autism and learning differences, because of the way the glands are being affected by environmental toxins. There really isn't anything "to be done" about it, except going to the leaders of industry and getting them to do things differently. It was an overwhelming evening. Sometimes what's important and galvanizing is really, really difficult, too. This is what isn't always addressed in the popular "green culture" publications!

But as a parent, I don't want to communicate to my children that the world is a scary place. If mama is upset, the whole household is upset. So I try to always maintain an emotional connection with them. To teach them to be conservationists as my parents taught me. And to keep doing my part to spread the word and make a difference.

Iroquois law counsels us to consider the impact of our decisions and interactions with others and with nature on seven generations down the line. Recently, while talking with my father about how we must act not just for our children but for their children's children and on from there, I wondered, how will we be judged? How will *I* be judged? My father, a financial advisor, said that as a new dad, he had thought about such things, too. Not a day went by when thoughts of his kids didn't motivate his actions. But he weighed his legacy, he said, largely in terms of wealth; he wanted to make sure he took care of his children financially.

I appreciate that idea. Yet, for me, and perhaps for many of my generation, I aspire to this legacy: *Your health is your wealth.* What I do in my life, the very values I try to live by, should connect to the kind of an environment and legacy of health I can leave for my children and, at least, for seven more generations. My father has come to appreciate this driving force, and not just because I badger him about it weekly.

When I look at my son, Luke, who at this moment is only a baby, I fantasize that one day he, or more likely his kids, will look at our generation and be glad that we took on the environmental challenges facing us. That they live on a cleaner, greener, healthier earth because of our actions.

Together we can make this come to pass.

CHAPTER I

Doing the Bump

PREPARING FOR BABY

Every parent is thunderstruck at the sight of his or her child-to-be on a sonogram. When I first laid eyes on my son, Luke, at about twelve weeks, I couldn't make out much of anything on the sonographer's screen. For a few moments, standing beside my wife, Jessica, who lay on the gurney, there was only the *swoosh, swoosh* of his heartbeat and a staticky gray background. Suddenly his spine came into focus. I was dumbfounded that his body, not much bigger than a peanut, already displayed such magnificent architecture, skull and organs so finely circumferenced, his whole neurological chassis maturing. At the same time, I was filled with a sense of his helplessness and fragility, his dependence on his mother for nourishment and safety.

Perhaps like no other time, pregnancy gives parents a chance to directly affect the health of their child. By making smart decisions about what you eat, drink, inhale, and absorb, you help stack the deck in your baby's favor, laying the foundation for many healthy years to come.

The umbilical cord is the life-sustaining vessel through which mom feeds her baby and removes waste, and across which vital hormonal signals pass. But just as the cord ushers growth-spurring nutrients and liquid to the baby during this critical period of organ and tissue growth, it also carries uninvited pollutants from mother's environmental exposure across the placental barrier.

This fact was starkly reinforced in a 2005 study by the Environmental Working Group (EWG) that examined cord blood from ten babies born in U.S. hospitals during a two-month span. What they found is heart-stopping: The cord blood contained an average of two hundred chemicals and pollutants commonly found in the home, including mercury, flame retardants, perfluorinated chemicals (from nonstick surfaces and carpet), plasticizers (PVCs), pesticides, and wood preservatives—many of which may cause cancer, are toxic to the brain and nervous system, and are linked to birth defects or abnormal development in animal tests. Because a fetus is so small, it is also much more vulnerable and less able to process and detoxify many of the chemicals it comes in contact with, leading to potentially irreversible effects. While the negative impact of many of these unwanted substances may be counterbalanced by good nutrition, reduced stress, and sleep, in the tug of war between healthy factors and risks, you naturally want to take whatever precautions you can for the sake of your unborn child.

200 **average number of chemicals and pollutants found in newborns' cord blood.** (Environmental Working Group, 2005)

Fortunately, there are things expectant moms can do to reduce their own exposures during pregnancy and to minimize a child's body burden from the start. Consider this five-step checklist for the health of the baby's first home: the womb.

Step #1. Eat Intelligently for Two

Your obstetrician will almost certainly urge you to make the following dietary adjustments: Cut out caffeine and alcohol. Eat a protein-rich diet with a variety of fruits, vegetables, and whole grains. Take prenatal vitamins with folic acid to protect against neural-tube defects and get enough omega-3. And for heaven's sake, don't smoke.

But he or she may not tell you about a few other strategies that support the health of your developing baby—eating a diet low in pesticides, artificial additives, preservatives, food colors, and other chemicals, as well as avoiding some of the major dietary sources of bacterial infection.

Go organic. During this time, eating lots of (and lots of different) fruits and vegetables provides important nutrients, so going organic—eating produce grown without chemical pesticides, fertilizers, or herbicides—makes particularly good sense. *You can lower your pesticide exposure by 90 percent* simply by avoiding the top twelve most contaminated fruits and vegetables, identified by the EWG.

If you stick with conventional (i.e., non-organic) produce, choose those with the lowest level of pesticide residue, and either peel or wash fruits and veggies with cold water and a gentle scrub brush to get rid of some of the microbes and chemical contaminants that may have hitched a ride in your grocery bag. (For more information about organic food, including a list of "The Dirty Dozen" fruits and vegetables, see Chapter 3.)

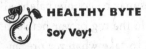

HEALTHY BYTE
Soy Vey!

Soy has lately gained status as a miracle food—and some experts have suggested that a high consumption of the hormonally active natural plant substances (phytoestrogens) present in soy explain the low incidence of estrogen-related cancers (like breast cancer) and heart disease in Asian women. But watch how much soy you eat during pregnancy: Studies suggest overexposure to phytoestrogens can be harmful to developing babies. Whenever possible, buy soy products—like tofu and soymilk—in their organic forms.

Mind your meat and dairy. Meat is a great source of protein and vitamin B_{12}, both important for pregnant women. However, really fatty sources contain dioxins and other nasty chemicals that can eventually be transferred to babies through breast milk—so slice off the fat and take your beef skinny. From now on, try to pick up organic meat and milk, minimizing your exposure to the antibiotics and hormones used in their production, all of which could be bad for mom's health—ergo, bad for baby's.

Find safer fish. The omega-3 acids in many fatty fish help spur baby's brain growth. But some fish, as you've no doubt heard, can harbor unhealthy pollutants. Many large species, including swordfish, king mackerel—and sorry to say, that sandwich staple, tuna—may contain elevated levels of mercury, which can upset normal fetal brain growth. Chunk light tuna is preferable to white albacore because it typically has lower levels of mercury (it comes from smaller fish). The EPA suggests that pregnant women can safely eat up to twelve ounces of chunk light tuna per week. Keep in mind that you'll want to weigh that number against your total fish consumption. Use the Environmental Working Group's tuna calculator at ewg.org/tunacalculator to find out how much might be best for you. To get more of those omega-3s that are so great for your baby's brain, pick smaller fish lower on the food chain, like sardines and mackerel. Or opt for nonfish sources (that are actually high in omega-3s) like flax seeds and walnuts.

Up to 600,000 estimated number of babies born each year with mild to moderate loss of IQ, due to in-utero exposure to methylmercury. Fish consumption is the likely culprit. (U.S. Environmental Protection Agency, 2004)

Farmed fish should also be consumed cautiously because the diets they're raised on tend to give them high levels of PCBs. These now-banned synthetic substances can cause long-lasting developmental delays in children exposed prenatally (and PCBs can linger in human fat for years). When ordering salmon, go wild—meaning wild Pacific. If you're unsure what type of salmon you're buying, ask your fishmonger or waiter. For a list of the best and worst of the sea, turn to page 74.

Watch your bac. Some types of bacteria pose particularly worrisome risks for pregnant women. Listeria is one. The CDC claims that pregnant women are *twenty times* more likely to become infected with the nasty microbe than nonpregnant adults. If mom-to-be does get sick from Listeria-contaminated food, the consequences for baby could be grave, ranging from miscarriage to infection in the newborn. The tricky thing about Listeria? Unlike many bacteria, it thrives at cold temperatures. Here are some strategies to prevent infection from these and other microbial critters, such as E. coli, salmonella, and toxoplasma:

- **Eat hard cheeses rather than soft.** The CDC recommends that pregnant women avoid soft cheeses such as feta, Brie, Camembert, and blue-veined cheeses. Pasteurized cheeses like cream cheese and sliced cheese are fine.
- **Don't cross-contaminate.** Raw foods and uncooked meat should not bump up against each other in the fridge or before cooking. After you handle raw meat, wash cutting boards, knives, counters, and hands in hot, soapy water.
- **Cook foods thoroughly.** Beef should be prepared medium-well to well done, with no pink showing; poultry should have no pink at the bone, with the juices running clear (165°F to 180°F); pork and ham should be well done.
- **Avoid raw eggs.** These can turn up in raw batter (no more licking the spoon!) or partially cooked egg dishes.
- **Ditch kitty litter duty.** Pregnant women should not change cat litter boxes. Toxoplasmosis, an infection from a parasite in cat feces, can threaten the health of an unborn child. If you must do it, wear gloves and thoroughly wash hands afterward, and don't breathe too close to the box.

Don't indulge junk food cravings. It can't be a surprise that many of the foods you crave during pregnancy, from nachos to candy bars, are not at all good for you, with empty calories and no nutritional upside. But another reason to sidestep processed food is that the preservatives, flavor enhancers, artificial colors, and other additives aren't great for a growing baby either. (Of course, hell hath no fury like a pregnant woman denied her craving. These are guidelines; you can go ahead and have that corn dog, just don't have one at every meal.) A few additives in particular to avoid, when possible:

- **MSG.** Monosodium glutamate is a flavor enhancer found in Asian cuisine and soups that can cause headaches and stomach upset. At high concentrations, it's also a neurotoxin (i.e., it kills nerve cells).
- **Artificial food coloring.** Fake coloring is present in many processed foods; the ones to steer clear of are blue 1 and 2, green 3, red 3, and yellow 6.
- **Artificial sweeteners.** Saccharine, the oldest fake sweetener, hasn't been shown to be safe for pregnant women. And aspartame has been linked to cancer in animal studies—prenatal exposure is most concerning.
- **Nitrites.** These food additives, normally found in hot dogs and sandwich meats, are possibly carcinogenic.

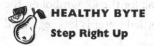

HEALTHY BYTE
Step Right Up

Sign up at healthychild.org for Healthy Child Healthy World's "First Steps to Healthy Babies" program, written by two of our science advisors, Dr. Harvey Karp and Dr. Sandra Steingraber. Parents can receive free monthly e-mail updates on their child's development and on how to protect them from environmental threats, during pregnancy and through the first two years.

Step #2. Get Clean Water on Tap

Obstetricians encourage pregnant women to stay hydrated, which promotes the flow of nutrients to the baby and also helps to keep amniotic fluid levels high. But concerns about unwanted junk in your water (specifically lead or chlorine) might give you second thoughts before turning on the faucet. Here is a quick reference list to ensure your water is clean. Skip to Chapter 7 for more information about each step.

Test your water for lead. This is especially important for those in older houses with lead-based pipes. Lead is one of the most toxic metals to children. See leadtesting.org.

Run cold water for a minute in the a.m. This will reduce lead that may have accumulated overnight.

Filter it. A basic tap filter or pitcher blocks the most common metals and microbes. You might also consider looking into a high-quality in-sink or whole-system filter. Remember to follow the manufacturer's recommendations for filter changes.

Cut back on bottled water. A recent study from Tufts University revealed some worrisome results from Bisphenol A (BPA), a commonly used chemical in plastic bottle manufacturing. Contained in clear polycarbonate plastics such as water and baby bottles, BPA can mimic estrogen and mess with reproductive growth. Look for the #7 symbol on the bottom of the bottle—and avoid it. Also, bottled water is less regulated than tap so there's no guarantee it's any cleaner.

Step #3. Be Naturally Gorgeous

Your skin is a porous organ, which means that a good deal of what you put on it may enter your body and be carried through the bloodstream, across the placenta. Many cosmetics, lotions, and shampoos contain harmful chemicals, including phthalates. Typically used to soften plastics, these chemicals also give personal care products a silkier feel, keep nail polish from chipping, and help fragrance last longer. Phthalates have been shown to alter male reproductive development in rodent studies, and preliminary research has suggested a link between high exposure to these chemicals in utero and male reproductive birth defects. Again, this is just one study, and the human health repercussions of these defects aren't well understood, but pregnancy is a time to be safe rather than sorry.

The EPA advises pregnant women to minimize their cosmetics and lotion use. To see how popular brands rank in safety and toxicity, check out the Environmental Working Group's "Skin Deep" report at ewg.org. (And for more information on all of these tips, see Chapter 4.)

But assuming you're not going completely *au naturel* for forty weeks, here are three grooming habits to give up while pregnant:

Nix the nail polish. Nail polish and removers are major sources of synthetic fragrances (ergo, phthalates); plus the solvents in these products may be particularly risky for pregnant women. Do you need more proof than the nose-scrunching scent? Fortunately, a few brands now make a phthalate-free polish. Gestating women are also advised not to get professional pedicures since the public foot-baths and sharp tools can harbor microbes. If you've just *got* to use regular nail polish, make sure you're in a place with decent air flow.

🌀 Expert Opinion 🌀
A Baby-Making Story
By Theo Colborn, president, The Endocrine Disruptor Exchange (TEDX), and professor, University of Florida, Gainesville

The making of a baby is like a fairy tale in some ways. Fairy tales are about giants and broken eggs and interesting animals, and things that no one will ever see. The story of the construction of a baby is about infinitesimally small things, so small that it is hard to believe, which makes it like a fairy tale. Instead of an egg breaking in the baby-making story, an egg, a single cell, begins to split over and over again until it forms a hollow ball of cells, at which time the cells begin to move about to form buds that become hands, feet, fingers, toes, arms, legs, and eventually organs and bones and muscle, and even a heart and a brain, which are all very real. That part of the story can be seen with microscopes and has been described with pictures in hundreds of textbooks in many languages.

When one asks, "What caused that single cell to split and keep splitting until it morphed into a baby?" the baby-making story begins to read like a real fairy tale. It is hard to believe that in the invisible universe where the egg is developing, there are hormones operating in the part-per-trillion range. And that each hormone is programmed to exert its influence on the construction of the baby only during rigid windows of time. No other period in the baby's life is as fragile as during those early days when its organs and brains are being constructed and programmed. And just as there are fairy-tale villains, there are many modern chemicals that can enter the womb environment and disturb its sacred hormonal balance.

Unfortunately, we live in a world where fantasy prevails. Anyone who believes that the womb environment is pristine believes in fairy tales. Anyone who believes that dangerous chemicals cannot invade the womb believes in fairy tales. And anyone who believes that everyday, low-dose exposure to industrial and agricultural chemicals cannot damage a developing baby believes in fairy tales.

Almost everyone becomes a baby-maker before he or she reaches old age. Even among those couples who prepare for parenthood and give it a great deal of thought, few are aware of the hazards posed to their product—their future child—by foreign chemicals in the womb. In "creating healthy environments for children," Healthy Child Healthy World is playing an important role in creating awareness of the vulnerability of the unborn child. Prevention is always preferable to treatment.

Practice safe scents. Fragrance-free products can reduce your exposure to phthalates, which aren't listed on the label but are often hidden in the word *fragrance*. Shelve the spritz, too—perfume is a major phthalate culprit.

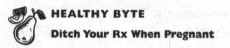

HEALTHY BYTE

Ditch Your Rx When Pregnant

If you use prescription skin medications, such as Accutane for acne or topical steroids for eczema, you'll want to give them up during pregnancy, as the CDC advises. Consult with your dermatologist and consider postponing plans for flawless skin. Anyway, pregnancy hormones wreak havoc with your face, causing skin to cycle between blemishes and that dewy glow.

'Do or dye. Some hair color products may contain harmful chemicals such as lead acetate and coal tar dyes. We don't have proof that hair dye is unsafe to use during pregnancy, but you're probably better off loving your roots for the rest of your term, and for as long as you're nursing. Highlighting products may be a better way to go, since the color generally doesn't come in contact with your scalp. Ask your stylist about the safety of the products at your salon, and try to make sure they don't contain lead or other heavy metals.

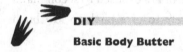

DIY

Basic Body Butter

Make this soothing cream with straight coconut oil (just scoop some into your hand) or by combining coconut oil and cocoa butter. Cocoa butter is great for dehydrated and cracked skin.

½ cup coconut oil

¼ cup cocoa butter

a few drops of essential oil (optional)

—*from* Home Enlightenment *by Annie B. Bond*

Step #4. Breathe Clean Air

Indoor air—the stuff we sleep in, play in, eat in; the air you might dare to call your own—can be far more polluted than the air outside; in fact, it's as much as *two to five times worse*, according to the EPA. Toxic chemicals, such as lead and pesticides, are found routinely in airborne household dust. Plus, many household products, from paints to glues to cleaning products, give off nasty fumes (known as VOCs, or volatile organic chemicals—more on these later) that place a burden on your fetus's health. In one study funded by Healthy Child, researchers at the Columbia University Center for Children's Environmental Health evaluated sixty newborns whose mothers wore portable air monitors during their last trimester and found that babies' DNA can undergo subtle damage by the polluted air their mothers breathe during pregnancy. During this period, stay on top of the following habits:

Banish smokers. Family members who smoke shouldn't do it anywhere near a pregnant mom, even when she's not there—the smoke clings to carpets and drapes and lingers for days. Tobacco smoke components, including nicotine, can quickly cross the placenta and lead to birth defects, while mothers who smoke or are exposed to secondhand smoke during pregnancy are more likely to give birth to low birth weight babies.

Clean green. During their last trimester, some women may find themselves in a Clean-up-this-dump-now-or-else frenzy. But conventional cleaning products can contain toxic chemicals such as ammonia, chlorine, formaldehyde, and artificial fragrances that may pose a risk if a pregnant woman is overly exposed. One study from the University of Bristol in the U.K. found that babies born to mothers who frequently used chemical-based cleaners while pregnant were more than twice as likely to develop breathing problems. Green household cleaners for every task are widely available, but tried-and-true Castile soap, baking soda, vinegar, and water are highly underrated. For more information on safe cleaning products and how to make your own, see Chapter 2.

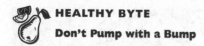

HEALTHY BYTE
Don't Pump with a Bump

Pregnant women should pull up to full-service gas pumps, if possible:
Pumping while pregnant can expose women and their fetuses to potentially hazardous fumes.

Freshen air naturally. Commercial air fresheners contain harmful volatile chemicals (VOCs). Even scented candles are a dubious option, as
some release harmful chemicals and some may even contain lead. Try
soy candles, which burn cleaner. Actually, growing indoor plants is the
greenest way to clear the air. For more information on improving indoor
air quality (and a list of plants), see Chapter 7.

Ventilate, ventilate, ventilate. For better airflow, throw open your windows as often as you can stand it to get a breath of fresh air and to release
the ongoing buildup of allergens and fumes from synthetic materials such
as carpet and furniture. If you live in a place prone to high levels of air
pollution, open your windows in the early morning and close them (or use
the air-conditioning) when air quality gets bad.

🌀 Expert Opinion 🌀
Choosing a Green Pediatrician
By Dr. Alan Greene, pediatrician and author of Raising Baby Green:
The Earth-Friendly Guide to Pregnancy, Childbirth, and Baby Care

A "green pediatrician" is aware of the environment's impact on a
child, and the child's impact on his environment. A growing body of
research attests to the powerful link between one and the other. The
food we eat, the products we put on our skin and use to clean our
homes, the toys children play with and put in their mouths—all of
these and more can affect the short-term and long-term health of a
child. A green pediatrician thinks about these issues. He or she is

interested in nutrition, exercise, and in working in concert with the
body's normal rhythms.

Here are five questions to ask your child's prospective, or even
current, doctor to help determine whether he or she is a green
pediatrician:

1. **Nutrition:** *How would you recommend my baby start solid foods?*
Or, for those with school-aged kids: *What do you recommend for
nutrition?*

Green pediatricians are excited about the great benefits provided by
good food, just as they are deeply concerned about the damaging effects
that additives and overly processed foods may cause.

2. **Ear infection:** *How do you treat it?*

Aside from a regular checkup, ear infection is the single likeliest
reason for a visit to the pediatrician. It's also tops in two other categories:
the reason for prescribing antibiotics and cause for surgery. A green
pediatrician wants to reduce the unnecessary use of antibiotics. Far too
often, the conventional pediatrician simply writes a prescription and
sends the suffering child home—even though, as both broader evidence
and my personal experience show, most ear infections go away on their
own, and in many situations will respond better *without* antibiotics. A
green pediatrician will often monitor and treat the child's pain and
discomfort while refraining from prematurely prescribing antibiotics.
Sometimes antibiotics are the best treatment, but by reserving them for
when they *are* appropriate, they will be more effective. Furthermore, a
child treated in this way is less prone to recurrences than one given
antibiotics early and too often.

3. **Eczema:** *How do you treat this?*

A conventional pediatrician tends to treat the symptoms, often with
steroid cream, while a green pediatrician looks first to determine what
might be triggering the eczema, an extremely common skin condition in
kids. Is it a food allergy? The home environment? The green pediatrician
might advocate a gentler approach, such as moisturizing the skin or

bathing the child in a different way. If those strategies don't suffice, then he or she might recommend medication.

In general, green pediatricians look for root causes. Another example: For ADHD, I'll frequently check serum ferritin levels (i.e., iron). Low total iron has been linked to ADHD in children, even in those with a normal finger-prick hemoglobin test. If subtle iron deficiency is present, I'll treat that.

4. **Child products:** *What kind of baby bottle do you recommend? Or: What's the best kids' shampoo? Sunscreen?*

Your pediatrician can be a valuable resource for recommending good products—and warning against bad ones. The answer to this question may shed light on the doctor's awareness of what's in the product (e.g., parabens or chemical preservatives in shampoos). It also provides an opening to discuss your concerns about other ingredients, and their relative benefit or harm.

5. **The doctor's own life:** *What's your favorite restaurant? What kind of car do you drive?*

For me, becoming a green pediatrician started with changes in my own life—namely, the illness of a family member—which then affected how I thought as a medical practitioner. The answer to this question may provide valuable insight into the doctor's worldview.

Though the doctor may not provide the "greenest" answers to your questions, *how* he or she answers is often just as illuminating. Willingness to engage in a dialogue may be the real hallmark of a green pediatrician. When choosing a doctor, you of course want someone steeped in science, and aware of recent literature and controversies. But you also want someone who articulates a point of view *and* desires to hear yours. I believe that teaching and inspiring one's patients, along with their families, about the value of nutrition, exercise, and attentiveness to environment may be of greater importance than the ability to write a prescription.

Step #5. Renovate Early—and Safely

Expectant parents tend to rush around in the weeks before baby's arrival regrouting bathrooms and giving everything a fresh coat of paint. This is not the time to pull a Bob Vila (unless you plan to move out while the reno's happening). Pregnant women and their fetuses are especially vulnerable to toxins from plaster and lead dust, particleboard (what most inexpensive furniture is made of these days), treated wood, and carpet fumes. In particular, avoid the urge to sand and scrape surfaces: The risk of ingesting chemicals, metals, and other unhealthy junk is huge. If at all possible, pregnant women should be banned from the job site and the area should be closed off from the rest of the house. Try to have your work done at least two months before your due date. Aside from all the dust that needs to get vacuumed and mopped up, fumes from new carpet, furniture, and paint (if it's the conventional kind) can take weeks to dissipate.

Paint a clean streak. Since the VOC fumes that waft from conventional paint (in part from the solvents that keep paints wet) can linger for weeks, and may be bad for baby's health, opt for one of the cleaner paint options now available. Low- and even no-VOC paints, which use water instead of petroleum-based solvents and contain no heavy metals or formaldehyde, are now widely available at home improvement stores. For more info on safe paints, see Chapter 9 and Healthy Resources at the back of the book.

Before you crack a single can, though, you'll want to be absolutely sure that your walls and trim are free of lead paint. Lead poisoning can pose harm to a child's developing brain, and babies can be exposed in utero. If you suspect you may have lead in your home—lead paint was banned in 1978, so homes built before then are more likely to harbor it—then check paint chips with a home-testing kit from your local hardware store (see page 225 for the most reliable ones) or have your home checked professionally. The National Lead Information Center provides a list of EPA-certified labs in your area (800-424-LEAD). If lead is found, you'll need to call in the pros.

Expert Opinion
Avoid Lead Exposure During Pregnancy
By Philip J. Landrigan, M.D., coauthor of Raising
Healthy Children in a Toxic World

I've seen some terrible cases of lead exposure during pregnancy. In these situations, pregnant moms and their partners decided to sand down old paint on window frames and doors because they wanted to make their homes safe and beautiful for their baby. Tragically, they didn't realize that the paint they were sanding had very high lead content. The sanding produced lead-contaminated dust, and the moms inhaled the dust. In one family, the mom developed a blood lead level of 45 mg/DL, an extremely toxic level. Lead passes easily across the placenta from mother to baby, and her baby was severely brain-damaged. The tragedy is that with proper information, this could have been completely avoided.

 # Parentblog
Keep the Pregnant Lady Away
By Tobey Maguire, actor, and Jennifer Meyer, jewelry designer

Jen: When I got pregnant, Tobey was incredibly involved. He came to every doctor's appointment, read books and articles, and helped me become conscientious about what to eat and what to avoid. We were so excited to do this together and do it right.

Tobey: One of the things I thought we were being really diligent about was deciding to paint Ruby's nursery months ahead of time. I'd been told about low-VOC paint and how it emits less fumes and fewer chemicals and is safer for pregnant women and kids. But when we got that layer of color up there, it still smelled—*really* bad. I was pretty frustrated, because we thought we were being so careful. *This* is the nontoxic paint? Then I did some research—all it takes is a little Googling—and I found out that there are lots of paints with *no* VOCs. But we'd already painted it with the next best thing.

J: We moved out of our house for two weeks because the smell was so strong, especially for me; when you're pregnant everything smells worse. And when we came home I didn't go near that room for another week.

T: She literally didn't go down the hallway.

J: Which was killing me because of course I was so excited to come home and see what my baby's room looked like!

T: I'm kind of strict about that stuff. Jen asked, "Come on, can't I just sneak a peek?" and I was like, *"Honey…"* So basically she didn't go in that room for a couple of months. I guess the moral of all this is to do your research first, use *no*-VOC paint, and get the job done well ahead of time. And keep the pregnant lady away from it.

J: That was really the first thing that brought to my attention that when it comes to your child, you've got to be involved in every little decision. The paint *seemed* like a little decision and it turned out to be a huge one.

T: The other thing we did was to rip up the carpet in Ruby's room. It can be expensive but we thought it was important to put down wood floors, because of the chemicals in carpet and the pollutants they trap.

J: We're really into clean floors. We don't wear shoes in our house because of all the stuff we track in. We have a basket of Crocs and slippers by the front door, and everybody has to take off their shoes— they're welcome to use anything in the basket. We get them washed and cleaned and keep them fresh for everyone.

T: People get used to it. And just to show it's not so extreme, I've been to other people's houses and worn my socks, and after being there for a few hours my socks are dirty. Like, *black.* In our house you can wear your socks all day—and they're white, because you're not tracking in a bunch of gunk.

J: And you feel comfortable having your baby crawl around on the floor.

T: Generally we just try to be aware of chemicals and waste. Ruby's toys are mostly cloth and wood, though inevitably you end up with some plastic.

J: I read the labels, and depending on the kind of plastic it is, I keep it or get rid of it. Tobey and I both come from the school of thought that she's just as well off playing with a pan and a wooden spoon. It's amazing how long she can be transfixed by something like a lemon. Instead of letting her chew on plastic toys because she's teething, we take tiny baby washcloths, dip them in water, and freeze them. It's her favorite teething toy rather than some gooey plastic thing.

T: We're also getting rid of all our water bottles. I drink a lot of bottled water—like, ten a day—and just recently we were like, okay, we've got to figure this out and get refillable glass or aluminum bottles.

J: We're making progress, but you have to move slowly so you don't get overwhelmed; so you don't think, "Oh my God, how can I make everything green, how can I make everything perfect and organic?" So when our paper towels ran out at one point, we replaced them with the recycled kind. Then we changed a few of our lightbulbs to CFLs. One step at a time. We eat organic food and go to the farmers' market. We decided to become more conscientious about our gas consumption and emissions, so we just bought a hybrid. You do the best you can. We use Seventh Generation diapers so we minimize our impact. I thought for a minute of trying cloth diapers....

T: I tried to encourage it. Jen said, "Okay, go ahead. But *you* clean it up!"

Build a healthy nursery. Since you're probably obsessing over what your baby's nursery will look like, if not already converting your home office into a cozy cocoon of pastels, here are a few health factors to keep in mind when outfitting a room:

Invest in healthy furnishings. Carpet, especially the newly installed stuff, can emit harmful chemicals from fibers, dyes, backing material, and flame retardants. Instead, go for hardwood floors (or bamboo or cork, two sustainable options) with organic or natural fiber area rugs. New furniture should, where possible, be made from untreated, natural woods, because fiberboard and pressed wood contain a mess of chemical finishes and glues. Hand-me-downs (or pieces you drag home from a tag sale) are great options for both rugs and furniture; just make sure old wood furniture isn't covered in lead paint.

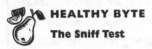

HEALTHY BYTE
The Sniff Test

It's not always possible to know what materials are in nursery products or how safe they are. One way to figure it out: Follow your nose. If the smell of a new piece of furniture, sheets, clothing, paint, or cleaning product is strong enough to bother you, it's strong enough to bother your baby, so don't put it in the nursery.

Opt for a natural crib mattress. A natural-fiber mattress is a splurge (often three hundred dollars or more) but arguably well worth it, given the many hours a day your baby will spend on it. Natural mattresses are usually made of organic cotton, which is grown without pesticides or herbicides. Conventional crib mattresses, on the other hand, tend to be covered in kid-unfriendly vinyl, stuffed with polyurethane foam, and treated with flame retardants—emitting fumes known to affect brain and nervous system development. Not something you really want your baby to lie on. (No matter what kind of mattress you get, make sure it's firm to protect against a heightened risk of SIDS, sudden infant death syndrome.) Crib sets, including sheets and bumpers, also come in organic cotton with no synthetic finishers. For more info, see Chapter 9; you'll find recommended brands in Healthy Resources.

DIY
Throw a Green Baby Shower

A green shower is a great way to exert some control over the influx of (often unwanted) plastic toys, not-your-taste clothes, and other gifts

from well-meaning family and friends. It's also a way to help introduce others—who may not yet be aware—to the benefits of organic and natural baby items.

Healthy Child and Seventh Generation threw a green baby shower for Sheryl Crow at her home in Nashville to welcome her son, Wyatt, into her life. Following was our master plan:

INVITATIONS

To save paper, invite guests via e-mail, like evite.com. Otherwise, seek out recycled content paper invites with soy-based ink. To pay it forward, consider Plant Me Seed-in-Paper Invitations: Guests can plant these in their yards when they're done. Find these at roundrobinpress.com.

SIPS AND BITES

Keep it pure and simple: Serve organic wine, beer, juice, and homemade nibbles. If you're having your event catered, choose vendors that work with local sources and organic ingredients.

TABLES

Avoid disposable paper or plastic table covers. If you're feeling ambitious, track down organic, fair trade, or vintage linens. Use your existing plates, flatware, and glasses. Anything to reduce waste is a bonus. (If you want to go the disposable route, you can find biodegradable flatware online.)

DECOR

Ask your florist to source flowers that are organically grown and, if possible, local. (Skip the floral foam and use flower frogs instead.) For an earthy vibe, scatter found objects (wood, pebbles, shells) and locally plucked greenery. Candles should be soy or beeswax to avoid harmful soot.

ACTIVITIES

Have guests decorate organic onesies using soy-based fabric paints. Or recruit them to write letters to Mom and baby by providing each place setting with a piece of recycled stationery and pen; then compile their output into a special book to be presented postshower.

GREEN GIFTS

Register at a green online baby goods store (find suggestions for an organic layette, wooden toys, and natural-fiber mattresses in the Healthy Resources section) and control the deluge of unwanted clutter. If it's your style, encourage friends who are parents to gift you with their gently used hand-me-downs. It's good for the planet; it's also good for your child, since conventional clothing that has been well washed loses much of its chemical finishers. Or give a donation to a great green organization—to help protect the legacy of a healthy world for the little one who will soon be born.

Think about Next Steps

As you count the weeks (okay, days . . . okay, *hours*) till your baby arrives, you're doubtless preoccupied with some of the nagging decisions of new parenthood: Which car seat? Which bottles? Do I really need a diaper system? Skip ahead to the following pages for more information on these topics:

- Diapers: cloth vs. disposable (pages 133–135)
- Baby-safe suds and creams (pages 108–111, 113–114)
- Natural layette and clothing (page 133–138)
- Safe baby bottles (page 99)
- Breastfeeding vs. bottle feeding (pages 99–101)
- What kind of water to use for baby formula (page 172)
- Binkys and teethers (pages 125–126)
- Car seats, high chairs, and other gear (pages 139–140)
- Lead- and PVC-free toys (pages 124–129)
- Nontoxic nursery furniture and décor (pages 31–32)

ONE STEP BEYOND
Come Up with a Green Birth Plan

There are many choices you'll have to make in the coming weeks, all of which affect your baby's exposure to the environment and harmonize your labor and delivery with ideals you espouse. Where do you plan to deliver your baby—at a hospital, in a birthing center, or at home? Who will be on your team—a medical doctor, doula, and/or midwife? Will you go for natural childbirth or will you opt for some level of medication, and at what point? And what will your baby's first meal be? Keep in mind that labor is full of surprises, and you have to be prepared to make adjustments during the big event. Still, it's good to have a clear plan of intention ahead of time, and to discuss it clearly with your caregivers—before the contractions begin.

CHAPTER 2

Cleanup Time

SAFE SUDS AND A GREENER CLEAN

W e keep so many of our cleaning products locked away under the sink and then proceed to spray and wipe and spill their contents all over the home. But that isn't all that's illogical about our pursuit of a totally sanitized home. (I'm one of four boys, so I know how messy kids can be!) How can cleaners be so, well, *unclean*?

The chemicals typically used in detergents, furniture polishes, floor waxes, window sprays, dish soaps, and tub and tile cleaners add up to a Who's Who of health hazards. Labels ominously marked WARNING or POISON suggest the immediate risks, should a child take a deep whiff or swig. But labels won't give you the full picture—of the known respiratory irritants, carcinogens, hormone disruptors, and neurotoxins associated with chronic and long-term effects—because these ingredients are part of secret formulas that manufacturers aren't required to divulge. (No wonder studies show that use of conventional household cleaning products is associated with chronic wheezing and asthma in children.) To top it off, when these chemicals are washed down the drain, any pretense to being

63

number of hazardous chemical products in the average American household, equal to roughly 10 gallons of hazardous waste. (Consumer Product Safety Commission, 2004) agents of "clean" disappears, as they can pollute our rivers and lakes, harming fish and wildlife.

Cleaning with nontoxic ingredients is one of the most important things you can do for your family's health. It's also one of the easiest. These days, eco-safe cleaning products can be found in abundance, at virtually every supermarket. And you don't have to be some kind of earth mother (or father) to make your own, using ordinary household ingredients such as baking soda, vinegar, and lemon. First, though, consider reducing some of the burden of cleaning altogether by leaving fewer things to clean.

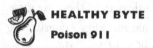 **HEALTHY BYTE**
Poison 911

Ten percent of all calls to the U.S. Poison Control Centers involve toxic exposure to household cleaners; of these, two-thirds concern children. Prominently display the number for the National Poison Control Center in your kitchen: 800-222-1222.

Step #1. Go Minimalist

You needn't whittle your life down to immaculate Zen spaces and sterile surfaces. But the payoff of a day (or three) spent decluttering your home will shock you. For one, dust—a fertile salad of mites, dirt, dander, and other particles—can contribute to allergies and asthma. It also encourages mold growth. Fewer surfaces equal fewer dust bunnies, less cleaning fluid, and less time and effort spent removing dirt. If you lack a slash-and-toss strategy, try these:

Institute a domestic clutter policy. Enforce daily decisions about which of the many objects you drag in get to stay—junk mail, knickknacks, food and toy packaging, shopping bags, kids' art projects—and which aren't worth complicating your life for even twenty-four hours. Keep a recycling receptacle by the door. Urge—better yet, insist—that family members pick up after themselves by scheduling an end-of-day cleanup time. Play fun music and set a timer for fifteen minutes. Make it a contest, or do it briskly enough that it's exercise.

Proceed room by room. It's better than randomly tossing clutter.

Part with those out-of-use possessions. You know you've hung on to things for reasons you can no longer rationalize. That lamp you haven't switched on in two years? *It is not your great-aunt Sally incarnate,* may she rest in peace. Seriously. You can give it to Goodwill without risking her ire from beyond the grave.

Resell, donate, recycle. If you're not a garage sale person, there are great Web sites where you'll find takers for your junk, including craigslist.org and freecycle.org. Or donate to charity. Simple rule: Something comes in, something goes out.

Step #2. Kick Your Chemical Habit

Switching to "chemical-light" cleaning products is extremely easy to do as a shopper; the tough part is breaking a habitual fondness for certain products—that one cleanser that actually gets your floors to wink back at you; the fabric softener that smells like childhood. Yet the more you learn about how these old reliables are bad for your family's health, the harder it becomes to continue using them.

Some of the most common and harmful chemicals include:

- **Ammonia.** A staple in bathrooms and kitchens for its ability to cut through dirt and grime and kill everything on contact. It's also a VOC, which is carried through the air to your nose as vapor, contributing to respiratory issues, perhaps worse.
- **Chlorine.** A component of many bleaching products, which can turn into highly hazardous chemicals when interacting with other substances. It's the number one household chemical involved in poisoning.
- **Phosphates.** Water softeners banned from laundry detergents in most states for their damaging effect on fish and freshwater systems but still found in some dishwasher and cleaning formulas.

- **Lye.** Used in drain and oven cleaners, detergent, pool cleaners, metal polishers, and soap, it's made from ash, and great at fighting grease and muck. Unfortunately, it can also irritate skin and eyes, and lye fumes can corrode respiratory passages.

These are just a few of the (known) *active* ingredients in cleaning products. Other potent chemicals—"inert ingredients," which usher the active ingredients to do their jobs—don't have to be listed on the label, because they're considered proprietary.

The label also won't clue you in to what's behind that pine forest or lemon aroma, which is injected into cleaning products to trick you into thinking they're as natural as the great outdoors. Synthetic fragrances, which are cocktails of up to hundreds of chemicals, are common triggers of allergic reactions and respiratory distress. So lose the artificial scents; your lungs and kids will be happier for it.

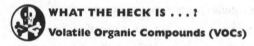

WHAT THE HECK IS . . . ?
Volatile Organic Compounds (VOCs)

VOCs are chemicals that are carbon-based and easily evaporate in the air—a phenomenon known as "off-gassing." Don't let the word *organic* fool you. VOC fumes come mainly from synthetic materials like plastic and polyurethane, paints and varnishes, and cleaning products. Whenever you smell something, whether fragrant (like the pine smell in cleaners) or putrid (like ammonia), it's likely a VOC. Not all VOCs are harmful, but some have been linked to everything from neurological and organ damage to cancer. Recent Australian studies correlated VOC exposure in the home with a higher incidence of asthma.

Virtually every conventional product you use now can be replaced with natural, environmentally sound alternatives available in any supermarket or home improvement store. Instead of chlorine or ammonia, green products' active ingredients are likely to be hydrogen peroxide or soap. Start with those you use most, like dishwashing and laundry detergents. Or kick off your conversion by getting rid of your most caustic

✂ Copy and Carry ✂
Green Cleaning Toolbox

Repeat this mantra: *I will no longer throw paper towels at my messes.** Instead, try reusable cleaning tools—all of which you probably own these.

Rags. Use strips of clothing, especially lint magnets like flannel and cotton. They should be broken out for different tasks (dusting versus wet-washing) and laundered regularly. Wearing an old sock on your hand also does the job.

Microfiber cloth. A new technology that uses no chemicals, microfiber cloths cling to dust and lint fiercely until washed.

Sponges. Choose cellulose because it's biodegradable. At least weekly— or when they start to smell—toss sponges in the dishwasher or microwave them. (If not washed frequently, they can harbor bacteria.) Replace often.

Broom and dustpan. Parents in love with their handheld vacs should consider a sweeping change because, while spot-cleaning a Cheerios trail is indisputably satisfying, it misses grit that can coat the floor and contribute to unhealthy air. If cared for, natural-fiber brooms last for years.

Mop. Keep a cellulose sponge mop for wet jobs, a microfiber one for dry. And forget the disposable mops-with-wipes: They're wasteful, expensive, and the chemicals on the wipes are nasty.

Bucket. Or two. Rinse after use to avoid the crusty riverbed look.

Scrub brush. Essential for scouring bathroom surfaces well enough so you don't yearn for harsh cleaning products.

Spray bottles. If you plan to make your own cleaning products, those with ounce labels are especially useful. You'll also need measuring cups, spoons, and glass jars with lids.

Old toothbrush. For scouring small or hard-to-reach spots.

HEPA Vacuum. The best way to clean carpet and upholstery. The most effective vacuums are equipped with a High Efficiency Particulate Air (HEPA) filter, which traps nearly all the tiny particles it sucks up; regular vacuums have a tendency to spew dust back out.

*Or at least consider switching to paper made from unbleached recycled materials. Look for the highest Post Consumer Waste (PCW) content that's Processed Chlorine Free (PCF).

household products—the ones you should be *sure* to avoid—like oven cleaners, drain decloggers, and toilet bowl cleaners.

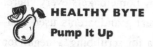

HEALTHY BYTE
Pump It Up

Look for cleaners that come in pump spray containers rather than aerosols, which produce a finer mist that's more easily inhaled.

When gauging ecological claims, watch out for "greenwashing" of ingredients. Terms like *natural* and *eco-friendly* should be backed up by specific ingredient information such as "no solvents," "no phosphates," "free from petroleum-based solvents, dyes, perfumes, and acids," or "biodegradable in seven days" (everything biodegrades eventually). While you're at it, buy cleaners in the largest available size, to save on packaging waste.

BURNING QUESTION
How do I get rid of bottles of cleaners I no longer use?

Since part of the motivation for switching from chemical to nontoxic cleaners is to reduce your impact on the environment, it can feel cringy (and hypocritical) to flush away these toxic brews. Some—including ammonia- and bleach-based cleaners, plus glass and tile cleaner—are generally safe to pour down the drain, but always do it separately and chase them with plenty of water (and *never* flush ammonia with bleach—it creates toxic fumes). If you have a septic system, however, save the chemical stuff for collection by the sanitation department. Same goes for the more caustic household products—oven, metal, and drain cleaners. Contact your local solid waste office to find out your own community's guidelines. For a thorough guide to hazardous disposal and other cleaning strategies, see *Green Clean* by Linda Mason Hunter and Mikki Halpin.

Step #3. Mix Your Own

Before the post–World War II household chemical revolution, when a gleaming kitchen became the pride of happy homemakers everywhere, most of our grandparents and all of our great-grandparents used relatively safe ingredients to clean: baking soda for scrubbing, vinegar for grease-cutting, vegetable soaps for bathing, citrus oils to fight odor, and hydrogen peroxide for its bleaching and bacteria-killing properties. Concocting your own formulas may seem daunting but it's actually very simple, not to mention inexpensive.

The Nontoxic Trio: Baking Soda, Soap, Vinegar

These three ingredients form the basis of many homemade cleansers and can be used alone or combined with other natural ingredients.

Baking soda. This multipurpose household staple softens water and neutralizes minerals, helping soap clean better (the two are often mixed together). Baking soda also absorbs odors, can be used as an abrasive for cleaning sinks and tubs, and helps to lift dirt away from whatever surface you're cleaning. A bit of baking soda on a sponge cleans up most countertop stains. *Washing soda* and *borax* are minerals related to baking soda, but stronger.

Soap. Soap cleans by dissolving oil that binds dirt to a surface. Opt for natural vegetable oil–based soaps, such as Castile or glycerin.

Vinegar. Available by the gallon at the supermarket, distilled white vinegar dissolves soap scum and mineral buildup and kills mold and bacteria, so it's especially effective on sinks and bathrooms. Its strong smell when poured disappears almost completely after drying. For a great glass cleaner, dilute with a 1:2 vinegar-to-water ratio.

By choosing from these natural ingredients, along with a few others— like *hydrogen peroxide*, a natural bleaching agent and antimicrobial, which is the active ingredient in many natural kitchen and bathroom cleansers;

lemon juice, a powerful acidic cleaner that fights mineral scum and grease; and *essential oils*, such as lavender and thyme, which add fragrance to cleansers and even boast antibacterial properties—you can clean just about anything.

Parentblog
A Little Help from My Kids
By Holly Robinson Peete, actress

My mother-in-law recently told me she thinks my kids ought to do more chores. "Give them some Lysol!" she said. I'm all for teaching kids responsibility but I told her I don't let them play with that stuff.

When my twins were born ten years ago they were both asthmatic. We used nebulizers; we tried aromatherapy, acupressure, acupuncture. They both ended up growing out of it, thank God. But now I'm dealing with my five- and two-year-olds, and you never know when something is going to trigger an attack.

Sometimes I wonder why this is happening to us. (I should mention that my oldest son, Rodney, is on the autistic spectrum, and there's lots of discussion in the scientific community about environmental causes for that, too.) I've noticed that strong chemical smells can trigger the twins' asthma. They're also both allergic to wheat and sometimes *that* causes it. To deal with their illness, we've had to make our home as healthy as possible, but it's been a steep learning curve.

For instance, one time we were fixing up a room and were about to lay down some carpet. It didn't occur to me that something could be wrong with that. I love that new carpet smell—who doesn't? But my nine-year-old daughter Ryan said, "You know, you need to be careful—there are so many chemicals in carpet!" She'd learned it in school. It's amazing to me that we're in an age where some kids are bringing back valid, valuable information about environmental health from school. I was like, "*Oh, my goodness*. I was going to put it down where my kids sit and my baby rolls around?!" I ended up putting down a bamboo floor, and we love it.

Then, when we renovated, we revamped the air-conditioning system so that it had a HEPA filter. It's helped to make our air healthier. We use humidifiers. We dust with microfiber cloths, which pick up every little speck. We have a HEPA filter on our vacuum; if you don't, you're pretty much just blowing dust back into the air and wasting your time.

For cleaning products, we use only nontoxic brands. With natural products, I feel more comfortable about my kids doing their chores, letting them clean the sink or wipe down the counter.

My next concern is their school environment, where most asthma attacks start. There's a tremendous amount of dust at their school. I've seen parents on cleaning duty but haven't noticed what cleaners they use. That's another thing to investigate. At least I can count on my kids to help me do it.

Here's an effective, all-purpose cleaner using ingredients found in most supermarkets that you can whip up in minutes.

All-Purpose Cleaner

Adapted from Annie B. Bond's Home Enlightenment

½ teaspoon washing soda
½ teaspoon liquid Castile soap
2 cups hot water
16-ounce spray bottle

Mix ingredients in spray bottle and shake gently. Use on counters, cupboards, or any surface. For tough dirt, leave the cleanser on for a few minutes before wiping it off. Can't find washing soda? Use 2½ teaspoons of borax instead.

Basic vinegar rinse to finish the job: Fill a squirt bottle with equal amounts white distilled vinegar and water. Add 15–20 drops of pure peppermint or tea tree oil (note that some botanical oils can be toxic if ingested). Shake. Great for floors, walls, windows, and for removing soap scum.

✂ Copy and Carry ✂

Your Under-sink Makeover

Compare the contents of a cabinet full of conventional cleansers with the greener, healthier cabinet. One-quarter the price, half the volume, twice the peace of mind. You do the math.

Old Cabinet	Green Cabinet
All-purpose cleaner	All-purpose nontoxic cleaner
Bleach	Baking soda
Carpet cleaner	Borax
Dishwasher detergent	Castile soap
Deodorizer	Dishwashing detergent (non-toxic)
Disinfecting wipes	Distilled white vinegar
Drain cleaner	Essential oils
Floor mopping detergent	Hydrogen peroxide
Floor wax	Liquid dishwashing soap (natural)
Furniture polish	Vegetable oil–based mopping liquid
Glass cleaner	**= $25**
Grout cleaner	
Liquid dishwashing soap	
Metal cleaner	
Oven cleaner	
Scouring cleanser	
Silver polish	
Soap scum remover	
Stain stick/remover	
Tile cleaner	
Toilet cleaner	
= $100+	

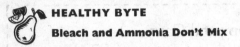

HEALTHY BYTE
Bleach and Ammonia Don't Mix

In case mom didn't tell you: Mixing bleach and ammonia releases a chlorine gas that can be fatal. The gas is so potent, in fact, it was used as a chemical warfare agent in World War I!

Step #4. Join the Clean Plate Club

Washing dishes—that inevitable daily chore and refuge for many a procrastinator—is one of the easiest places to start greening your cleaning. Use an eco-friendly, nontoxic brand of dishwashing soap, available in any grocery store, or make your own from Castile soap and water. More dish on getting plates spotless:

Washing by hand. Rinse dishes as soon as possible (so much for procrastinating) so there's less grit-chiseling later. Instead of letting the water gurgle ceaselessly down the drain, fill two basins or sinks, one for washing, one for rinsing. Clean glass or crystal first (vinegar in the rinse water prevents spotting), then plates, then silverware. Before washing pots and pans, by sprinkle baking soda on encrusted food. For cast-iron, forgo soap altogether (and definitely don't soak or pans will rust), then rinse, wipe down, and re-season with vegetable oil.

Using the automatic dishwasher. In the epic, age-old debate—Which uses less water, automatic dishwashers or hand washing?—the machines (at least those that carry the EPA's Energy Star label) now consistently triumph. Skip conventional detergents, which may contain phosphates, and opt for chemical-free, biodegradable alternatives. For best energy savings, pack your machine fully, and run the dishwasher on energy saver or economy mode.

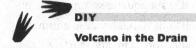

DIY

Volcano in the Drain

Drain decloggers are among the most toxic household products: harmful to your health, your pipes, your septic tank, and our water supply. Kids will love this homemade, natural drain cleaner, best used preemptively every couple of weeks rather than after the drain has a nasty backup:

Pour one cup baking soda down the drain, then one cup vinegar with a few drops of food coloring. Once the bubbling and frothing (and squealing) cease, pour in a pot of boiling water. Bottoms up.

Step #5. Banish Antibacterials

Antibacterial soaps and disinfectants have attained almost mythic status in American households, likely because of their promise of hypercleanliness and microbial eradication. Yet a growing number of health professionals warn that our efforts to rid ourselves of all kinds of germs, and the proliferation of these antibacterials, do us more harm than good.

For one, some bacteria are naturally beneficial parts of our body's ecosystem, so killing them can damage skin and weaken the immune system. A current theory—"the hygiene hypothesis"—asserts that our efforts to live in an ultra-clean environment have contributed to the alarming rise in asthma and allergies. In effect, by *not* challenging our immune systems with germs, our body's defenses may shut down and lose the ability to respond effectively when confronted with a real invader.

For another, this constant assault by antibacterial products is thought to contribute to the breeding of "super germs," or bacteria resistant to disinfectants and drugs—which makes the whole point of getting "clean" pretty much moot, if some germs are returning stronger than before.

Triclosan is the main ingredient in most antibacterial and disinfectant soaps and sprays; it's related to one of our deadliest pollutants, dioxin, which can form when triclosan is mixed with water and exposed to sunlight. By washing triclosan down the drain, we doubtless harm the environment, and it has been shown to disrupt aquatic systems. The human health effects of triclosan aren't well known, but because antimicrobials leave a residue on skin and surfaces that have been cleaned, they practically single out young children, who tend to suck on their fingers. Learn more by going to beyondpesticides.org and searching *triclosan*.

66

percentage of 139 streams sampled in 30 states that were found to contain disinfectants.

(United States Geological Survey, 2002)

For the average home, plain old soap and water are just as effective for eliminating germs. And studies show that some botanical oils, such as lavender and thyme, contain strong antibacterial properties.

DIY

Homemade Soft Scrubber

Use this on countertops and the sink; it's also great for bathtubs and shower stalls. Make only as much as you'll use in one cleaning session, because it dries out quickly.

½ cup baking soda

liquid soap or detergent

5–10 drops pure antibacterial essential oil, such as lavender (optional)

Place baking soda in a bowl. Slowly pour in liquid soap, stirring constantly, until consistency resembles frosting. Add essential oil, if desired. Scoop creamy mixture onto a sponge; scrub the surface, then rinse.

—*from* Home Enlightenment *by Annie Bond*

Scrub in (and out). The important thing is not the type of soap you use, or whether or not it prevents the spread of bacteria and viruses. It's how you wash your hands, and how often. Wash before and after preparing food; before eating or handling contact lenses; after changing a diaper, petting animals, sneezing, coughing, or using the toilet; and whenever hands come in contact with bodily fluids. Teach your child to rub both sides of the hands, between fingers, around cuticles and under fingernails. She should rub for as long as it takes to sing the alphabet song. The physical act of washing with soap and water removes all kinds of microorganisms, including the viruses that cause colds and the flu (which, cruel irony, aren't even knocked out by antibacterials).

275
number of active ingredients in antibacterial products classified as pesticides.
(Environmental Protection Agency, 2007)

Clean surfaces with hot, soapy water. Scrub surfaces well to loosen bacteria, which can form a slimy layer resistant to detergent alone.

Disinfect naturally. Clean those objects that come into contact with raw meat, fish, or eggs, such as plastic cutting boards, utensils, and counters, with a good scrubbing and lots of soap. You can safely sanitize surfaces by first wiping them clean with vinegar, then using a spray cleaner with hydrogen peroxide. If the hydrogen peroxide doesn't bubble on contact, you need to get a fresh bottle.

HEALTHY BYTE
E-lemon-ate Your Dirty Nuker

Deodorize your microwave by placing lemon slices in a microwave-safe cup with at least eight ounces of water. Heat on high for three minutes. Let sit for three more minutes without opening the microwave door. Remove the cup and wipe down the inside of the microwave.

Step #6. Wipe Away Mildew and Mold

As the third of four boys, I was gifted with the job of cleaning the bathrooms at home, where mildew blossomed from nonstop shower taking (we all played sports). Scrubbing the shower stall with standard cleanser made me woozy from the gases, which is no surprise: Just fifteen minutes cleaning scale off of shower walls could subject a person's lungs to an amount three times the "acute one-hour exposure limit" for glycol ether-containing products set by the California Office of Environmental Health Hazard Assessment. But the alternative is lousy, too—mold and mildew spores are one of the leading causes of asthma and allergies. Some lessons I learned:

Act fast. The instant you discover mold and mildew, identify the moisture source and stop it. It's pointless to clean mold if it's going to creep right back. Got a leak in your wall, basement, or elsewhere? Seal it or get it repaired ASAP. (For a serious problem, such as the notorious "black mold" that grows in damp drywall, call in the professionals, such as Disaster Restoration at gotmold.com or 866-GOT-MOLD.)

Stay high, stay dry. Bacteria and fungi thrive in moist, warm places; they'd send them cards and flowers if they could. So keep surfaces moisture-free and ventilate well. Laundry baskets should be able to breathe. Crack the window or hit the vent when cooking or bathing. If you've got a soggy area, use a dehumidifier to reduce moisture.

De-mold safely. It's a myth that you need chlorinated bleaches, ammonia, or other chemically potent mold and mildew cleaners to obliterate spores. For problem areas, wear gloves and a face mask (spores can be inhaled) and use a stiff bristle brush or toothbrush, a non-ammonia detergent (such as borax, hydrogen peroxide, or tea tree oil), and hot water. Or spray with a solution of a half cup of vinegar to a cup of water.

 DIY

A Little Help Around the House

Keep on hand a couple of spray bottles filled with soapy suds (a little Castile soap mixed with tap water). Kids love to go around wiping up surfaces, floors, you name it, while "helping" Mom or Dad. Sure, you may have to secretly re-clean after them, but it's worth it—growing up cleaning teaches kids a good habit, meaning less work for you down the line.

HEALTHY BYTE
Freshen Up Your Air

The air in your home will be so much cleaner if you cut back on chemically laced household products. Other ways to improve indoor air quality (see Chapter 7 for details):

Open windows. Keep the fresh air flowing—especially while you clean. Even a few minutes a day can significantly improve indoor air quality.

Deodorize naturally. To eradicate the pungent memory of last night's fish dish, use only products scented with essential oils or other botanical fragrances. Vinegar is a natural deodorizer (it stinks when you first spray it, then the smell dissipates); wipe down the smelly or sticky areas with a vinegar solution or just place a small bowl of vinegar in the room.

Skip the plug-ins. Those socket-bound air fresheners may make the house smell pleasant but—you guessed it—they give off synthetic fragrances that aren't benign when inhaled. To scent your home without the chemicals, add citrus peel, cinnamon, cloves, or any herb or flower petals to a small pot of water. Simmer on the stove.

Step #7. Tread Lightly (and Cleanly)

You'd never lick a shoe (you wouldn't, would you?) yet your child crawls on the floor and sucks her fingers. So inviting into your home the dirt, chemicals, bacteria, feces, lead dust, pesticides, allergenic dust, animal dander, and other domestic interlopers carried underfoot would seem unwise. The professional cleaning industry estimates that 85 percent of the dirt we bring into our homes enters via our shoes or our pets' paws.

What's more, carpets trap chemicals that originate inside the house as well as those tracked in from outdoors. So a great place to begin childproofing your home is with the carpets and floors, since young kids, being naturally low to the ground, use the floor as their primary play space.

Hard Surfaces

Use a doormat. According to the 1991 EPA report fittingly called the "Door Mat Study," lead-contaminated soil from outside causes most of the lead dust inside homes built after 1978. The study also notes that wiping shoes on a mat and removing them at the door can cut lead dust by an impressive 60 percent. Limiting what you track in can also reduce exposure to pesticides and other pollutants. Even better than using a doormat, leave your shoes at the door. If you're uncomfortable making people shed their shoes, keep a few pairs of slippers or socks in a basket near the entrance.

Spot-clean. Wipe up spills as they happen and sweep away dirt or grit underfoot with a broom or microfiber mop.

Hop on a mop. Floor cleaners come in a range of specializations for different surfaces—from wood to vinyl to tile. They may purport to do different things, but they're all designed to leave behind a glossy sheen once the liquid evaporates, and that chemical layer is what your kids slide around on and come in contact with.

In truth, plain soap and hot water gets your floors as clean as conventional products. Try a natural, biodegradable store-bought option. Or combine a quarter cup of vegetable oil–based soap with a half cup of distilled vinegar and two gallons of hot water. For wood floors, substitute a teaspoon of glycerin for the vinegar. You can also polish floors with linseed oil, available in home improvement stores.

Carpets and Rugs

Conventional carpet cleaners, particularly the aerosol kind, spew chemicals into the air for all-too-easy inhalation. But carpeting itself presents a significant health issue. Synthetic carpets contain chemical stain repellents and mildew treatments, not to mention toxic chemicals in the glue binders and rubber cushioning, which can release fumes ("off-gas") for months.

Wool or other natural-material carpeting such as hemp, jute, or coir are healthier options. Also, try these healthy maintenance tactics:

Clean up stains. As with hard surfaces, blot spills as they happen. Use nontoxic cleaners or see our spot-cleaning guide on page 55.

Deodorize naturally. Sprinkle baking soda on the carpet and let it stand for fifteen to thirty minutes before vacuuming.

Vacuum regularly. This is especially important if there are asthma sufferers around. Ideally, use a machine fitted with a HEPA filter to trap small particles that otherwise blow back into the room through the walls of a regular vacuum bag.

Steam clean occasionally. Professional rug cleaners tend to use the harshest of chemicals to treat carpet. You can do the cleaning yourself— a nontoxic version—by renting a steam cleaner from a local home improvement store or supermarket and pretreating spots with lemon juice and one-eighth of a cup of liquid soap to two gallons of hot water. Repeat until water comes up clear. Important: The rug or carpet should be thoroughly dry before children are allowed back in.

Use a dehumidifier. If your carpet is in a damp room, this machine will discourage mildew growth.

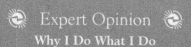

Expert Opinion
Why I Do What I Do
By Jeffrey Hollender, president and chief inspired protagonist, Seventh Generation

People occasionally ask me why I do what I do. There are lots of answers but the truest is that I've got children. Once you bring a child into being, you view your days through a different lens. The things you do are not the things you've done. The things you want are not the things you wanted before.

Many years ago, my son Alex, who was then five, fell ill. A rough spring was followed by a worse early summer. He wasn't so much sick as simply sickly, and as my wife and I looked on helplessly, he seemed unable to get better. The doctors couldn't find anything wrong, but something was very clearly not right. The only thing we could pinpoint with any confidence was our growing fear as we watched him slip downhill.

One day, while I was working out of state, my wife called me, frantic: Alex was having trouble breathing. I could actually hear him in the background, gasping for air. While my wife rushed him to the nearest hospital, I did what any father would do. In utter panic, I raced to the airport at an outrageously illegal speed, threw every credit card I had at the charter desk, and actually hired a private plane to fly me to a tiny airport within sprinting distance of the hospital.

By the time I arrived, Alex was recovering from what had been diagnosed, to my shock, as an asthma attack. Asthma? *My son has asthma?* It was awful to think about, but at least now we had an answer, unsettling though it was. Armed with this knowledge, we went to a specialist in New York City, who proceeded to give us a long lecture on how the key to treatment wasn't drugs but creating a healthy home. My wife and I listened dutifully as the doctor went on about things like toxic dust, household cleaners, and indoor air pollution.

Today, Alex is in his first year of college. We'll never know what triggered his asthma, but we know what steps we can take to help prevent future attacks and keep him safe. We know how to create that healthy home the doctor spoke about, and we have.

What I want is for everyone else to know, too. Because so many people simply don't. They have no idea how truly dangerous so many of the chemicals and technologies are that we surround ourselves and families with. Through no fault of their own, most people are largely oblivious to the hazards present in a bottle of conventional household cleaner or the toxic chemicals in the vapors created by something as ordinary as a dishwasher.

People just don't realize that many of the things surrounding them are turning their homes into toxic sinks in which the air is two to five times more polluted than the air just outside. Most of all, they don't realize what all these things can do to the most vulnerable and defenseless among us.

I don't want anyone else to feel what I felt on that scary summer day. I don't want another child to suffer. From where I sit, I can see the place where those things never happen. I can see a world that's safe, clean, and healthy, one that nurtures life instead of harming it, and we're going to get there.

✂ Copy and Carry ✂
Carpet Spot-Cleaning Guide

Mineral water makes an excellent stain remover. Use a clean terry cloth to blot out spots right after the spill. Be persistent—not all of them come out easily.

For fruit and wine spots. Blot with a towel and add cold water, continuing to blot. For red wine, use salt or club soda.

For grease. Use boiling water followed by dry baking soda.

For blood. Use cold water or hydrogen peroxide or try a paste of cornstarch or corn meal with water. Allow to dry and brush away.

For rust. Saturate with lemon juice and rub with salt.

Step #8. Sort Your Laundry

Death and taxes . . . and laundry. Just when we finish a load, another one piles up. The average American household does four hundred loads of laundry a year—meaning huge amounts of water and energy used, and chemicals washed down the drain that pollute the water system.

What's more, our lust for clean laundry exposes everyone to an excessive onslaught of chlorine bleach, optical brighteners (which may promote allergic reactions), artificial fragrances, and numerous other harmful chemicals too depressing to list here. Happily, there are healthier alternatives—and your clothes will look no less bright for soaking in them:

Use nontoxic laundry liquid. It contains no petroleum products, phosphates, chlorine, or synthetic toxic fragrances and dyes; you can find a variety of brands at most supermarkets.

Skip the chlorine bleach. Yes, linens get sweaty and sometimes little kids pee on them. But chlorine, bleach's active ingredient, is a powerful disinfectant that's harmful if inhaled, that weakens certain fabrics, and that can react with organic materials in water to form toxic by-products. To brighten safely, hang sheets outside on a sunny day or, in lieu of ordinary bleach, use a hydrogen peroxide–based solution, or a cup of vinegar per load. Maybe your white sheets will no longer blind you with their brightness but to breathe easier seems a worthwhile trade.

Replace your chemical fabric softener. Substitute with baking soda. Just one-half to three-quarters of a cup of it tossed into the wash leaves clothes soft and fresh-smelling.

Wash less. Seriously—if there's no smell or stains . . . why? All that energy, water, time, when no one will really know the difference?

ENERGY SAVER
Chill Out
Ninety percent of the energy used for washing clothes goes to heating the water. Switch the setting from hot to warm and cut your load's energy consumption by half. Also, electric dryers are often the top energy suckers in a home. Clean out lint after every use to keep hot air moving efficiently, and dry full loads. If you're inclined, line-dry some of your duds, especially towels and sheets, which will radically reduce your carbon footprint on the environment (not to mention shrink your utility bill).

HEALTHY BYTE

The Wrinkle in Dry-Cleaning

If you dry-clean lots of clothes and remove the plastic shroud in a bedroom or well-trafficked hallway, then you're all inhaling "perc" (perchloroethylene, also known as PCE), the highly toxic and carcinogenic dry-cleaning fluid. Amazingly, despite the EPA's listing perc as a hazardous air pollutant in 1997, four of five dry-cleaners still use it.

Though some manufacturers' labels insist on "dry-clean only," many clothes can be hand- or gently machine-washed and line-dried, especially woolens and silks. For those clothes that do require professional cleaning, try to find a cleaner in your area that offers "wet cleaning," which uses no solvents or toxins. (See epa.gov/dfe/pubs/garment/gcrg/cleanguide.pdf for state-by-state listings.)

If you continue to dry-clean, reduce your perc exposure by removing the plastic liners outdoors or in the garage, and let clothes air out for a day or two. *Then* put them in your closet.

Step #9. Bug Out Safely

Insects are the most diverse group of animals on earth, with more than a million known species, so even the most meticulous housekeeper will occasionally have a bug problem. Wherever there's food, moisture, or clutter, you can pretty much guarantee that insects will move in.

You could take a can of bug poison to wipe out each infestation, of course, but do you really want to spray your home with a pesticide, one that's formulated to kill small creatures, in areas where your own small creatures play, eat, and breathe? Eventually these poisons leach into soil, plants, water, and our bodies. Plus, spraying with conventional pesticides is only a quick fix, since it usually doesn't eliminate the source of the problem.

There is a healthier option. Called Integrated Pest Management (IPM), it's an approach used increasingly by gardeners and pest professionals who have learned that chemical controls have their price, including waning effectiveness, since bugs develop resistance with overuse. The main tenet of IPM: A home will never be 100 percent pest-free. And, in fact, a home that's 90 percent bug-free is better than one that's completely bug-free but which has replaced unwanted insects with toxic residues. Truth is, nature has a way of bypassing the chemical barriers that are erected. So the first step for the squeamish: Get over your fear of the little spider setting up house near your basement door. Some bugs are your friends. Here are some natural strategies for reducing the ones you don't want:

Prevent pests from thriving. Don't be so hospitable! Deprive them of food, water, and shelter so they look elsewhere to live. Clean up food and drink spills immediately. Seal food in airtight containers. Remove clutter, such as newspaper stacks, where bugs like to hang out.

Maintain your home. Upkeep is crucial, especially in damp and porous areas. Repair leaky plumbing, which quenches pests' thirst and moistens their air. Caulk up cracks and block holes both inside and outside the house to bar critters entry and freedom of movement. And use barriers, such as window screens, to prevent insects from slipping in.

Use the food chain. Spiders are natural predators of most pests, and the majority are completely harmless, so allow some of them to become extended houseguests. You can also enlist other predatory insects (ladybugs, lacewings) and birds to feast on pests by creating a hospitable habitat in your backyard.

Try natural bug repellents. Many ordinary household ingredients repel pests of all kinds. Beyond Pesticides (beyondpesticides.org), a nonprofit group that promotes safe alternatives to toxic pesticides, offers a guide. To be rid of unwanted insects, try a few of these tricks:

- **Ants.** Sprinkle paprika, dried peppermint, peppermint essential oil, or powdered soap where ants invade. Boric acid, a mineral with insecticidal properties, may be injected into cracks and small openings; when insects walk through these it sticks to their legs and eventually gets eaten, starving or dehydrating them. (Note: Only use boric acid, which can be harmful if ingested, where kids and pets can't get to it—behind refrigerators, under sinks and stoves, etc.) You can also remove the food the ants are coming for, wait twenty minutes, then clean up their trail with vinegar and plug up the hole they marched out of.

- **Cockroaches and silverfish.** Use boric acid—again, applied only in places safe from kids and pets—or silica gel (without chemical additives). Don't leave water standing or leave bar soap out—they eat it!

- **Dust mites.** Use mattress and pillow encasings that are impermeable to dust mites; stay away from feather comforters, feather pillows, and stuffed animals (if your child is asthmatic, it may be wise to keep stuffed animals, a paradise for dust mites, off the bed); wash bedding in hot water; clean frequently using a vacuum fitted with a HEPA filter.

- **Moths.** Replace mothballs—which contain naphthalene, a carcinogen—with cedar chips. (Note: In some children, cedar can trigger asthma.) Put the mixture in potpourri bags to avoid a big mess. For pesky moths that thrive on pantry foods, get sticky-surface cupboard moth traps that are nontoxic and free of pesticides. (See Healthy Resources.)

- **Rodents.** Plant sprigs of lavender or mint around your house; in strategic areas (basement, kitchen), place pieces of cardboard saturated with essential oil of peppermint. Cut back tall grass and brush from around the foundation and clean up rotting produce from the garden.

Call in the pros. If it's finally time to hand the job over to a professional, look for an IPM practitioner. Beyondpesticides.org has regional listings. Many firms merely talk a good game on IPM. If you're searching for a pest company but don't have a reliable reference, ask lots of questions to know exactly what they're using.

Parentblog
Use Your Network
By Courteney Cox, actress

Among my friends, I'm the "green" novice. I was born and raised in Birmingham, Alabama, which wasn't as progressive a city as Los Angeles. There wasn't any real awareness, in my house at least, about harm from pesticides or lead paint or about anything green. After I moved to California, though, I ended up surrounding myself with people who were very informed about those issues and who since then have taught me a lot. My friends will say, *Courteney, there's a great new car seat that's the safest one on the market.* Or, *I found some really cute organic cotton pajamas for Coco—they're better for the environment and better for her health.* My friend Laura turned me on to goat's milk—it can be easier for some kids to digest than cow's milk. I'm just learning this stuff, but I'm lucky that they pass along their wisdom.

That's not to say that I follow whatever they say. I don't take it as far as many of them do, because it's not like everything in my home that's *not* green is unsafe. I just try to make sure my house is filled with healthy products—organic food, nonchemical shampoos, body lotions, and cleaning products. Don't get me wrong, though: I still won't get rid of my Windex.

Being a parent is tough enough. We all do the best we can and no one wants to feel forced into changing their habits. You have to come to it in a comfortable way, but if you keep an open mind, and a network of smart and well-informed friends, relatives, and specialists that you can turn to for information, it will make that learning process a pleasure.

Step #10. Detox the Garage and Basement

Which areas of the home contain the most dubious, potentially dangerous substances? The garage (which *is* just a *b* short of "garbage") and basement tend to be repositories for mystery bottles and cans, containing

hazardous chemicals that should be kept out of children's reach, like motor oil, antifreeze, paint, turpentine, insecticide, rat poison, etc. These
spaces are dark and dirty, moist and moldy, but you can significantly reduce, if not eliminate, the dampness, dust, and other allergens that exist
there.

Conquer dust and mold. Spring-clean (or anytime-clean) your garage
and basement, getting rid of cobwebs, dust balls, and other allergen col-
lectors. If the walls are made from drywall and the room tends to be
damp, consider having it tested for mold: Drywall is a magnet for mold
spores that contribute to asthma and other respiratory infections. Run a
dehumidifier occasionally, especially after a heavy rain. (For more information on mold testing, see Chapter 7.)

Dispose safely. Hazardous waste can't be left in the street or in a
Dumpster. If you have a small amount of paint left in a can, open the
lid, let the liquids air-dry in a well-ventilated area, wrap the whole thing
in newspaper, and put it out with the trash. Oil-based paint and full
cans of latex, however, must be taken to a waste collection center.
Other flammable liquids—motor oil, turpentine, varnish—must be dis-
posed of responsibly. Different states and counties have different laws.
Visit earth911.org or call your local sanitation department to find out
what's permissible where you live, and for tips on recycling and disposing of all sorts of chemical waste and materials like computers.

Store smartly. Keep toxic substances (such as those mentioned above)
in their original containers up on a high shelf, far from little hands;
never reuse containers. House these products in a dry, cool (not freezing) area, away from heat, flames, or sparks. If your garage shares walls
or ceiling with living spaces, consider erecting a foil vapor barrier to
block the passage of moisture and fumes into your home. Another reason for an extra barrier: It blocks pollutants your engine emits after the
car is turned off.

ONE STEP BEYOND

Rid Yourself of Chemical-emitting, Gunk-collecting, Wall-to-wall Carpeting. Several carpet makers offer reclamation programs so you don't overtax landfills. For example, Los Angeles Fiber (lafiber.com) will pick up an old carpet from your home (you pay only freight), then recycle and convert the material into carpet cushion.

Green-clean your car. Use the same nontoxic upholstery and hard-surface cleaners as you do for your home.

Enlighten your school, day-care center, or community group. Encourage them to swap unhealthy chemical cleaners for nontoxic ones.

CHAPTER 3

A Clean Plate

CHOOSING, EATING, AND STORING
HEALTHIER FOOD

L ike every American kid, I read the cereal box while eating breakfast. I wanted to know what I had to do to win the prize, or what was in the flakes I was shoveling into my mouth. In fact, I can't remember *not* being into nutrition. When I was eight, my soccer coach ordered us, "Before the game, eat bananas!" I didn't understand why at first, but then I began to realize that my performance and mood seemed to depend on what I had just eaten. I started to wonder, *What do I need to eat to succeed?*

Years later, when I worked with kids struggling with developmental and health problems, I'd ask their parents to consider a version of that question. *What does my child need to eat to be smart, energetic, healthy?* The healthier and more appropriate the food we consume, the more likely the positive outcome. To dads I'd sometimes point out that they would never put bad gasoline or inferior engine parts into their car. Why do the equivalent with their kids?

At Healthy Child, we're concerned about children's nutrition, especially given the exploding juvenile obesity rate in the United States. But now dietary science is teaching us that "You are what you eat" goes way beyond ensuring that kids eat balanced meals. Today we're learning more about food-borne health risks, such as artificial additives, not to mention pesticides, hormones, antibiotics, and genetically altered foods.

Parents aren't going to win every battle; kids are going to eat gummy bears at birthday parties and chow down on hot dogs at ball games. The keys are moderation and judgment—and learning to ask, *Is there a healthier option? One that's less processed?* Incidentally, I think it's also important to ask questions like, *Where was this food made? Was it picked in, say, Chile or New Zealand and shipped thousands of miles to my supermarket?* and *Does that make sense for the environment?*

The abundance and variety of food these days can make you dizzy. Fortunately, more mainstream companies are cleaning up their act, and organic product sales are increasing by more than 20 percent each year. To pick healthier foods for your family, and to help forge a greener future for food production, here are ten steps to consider when shopping for it, preparing it, and yes, eating it.

Step #1. Crack the Label Code

Food labels often seem as if they're designed to frustrate and mislead. You know the feeling: Somewhere after high-fructose corn syrup (a sweetener) and before potassium sorbate (a preservative), your eyes cross. So you either put the can back on the shelf or just drop it in your cart with a resigned shrug.

Ingredients are listed in order of their weight contribution. If you don't recognize the first few, it's a red flag that the food is probably not supernutritious (the exception may be fortified cereal, whose unpronounceables could be vitamins). If one of the first two ingredients is a sweetener—either sugar or that ubiquitous high-fructose corn syrup— you might as well eat it for dessert.

Foods will often tout their health benefits—"organic" or "low-fat"— while glossing over the fact that they contain sugars or other additives. Like so much regulation in our country, our government's oversight of food is a spotty affair and often lets claims that manufacturers make about their products go unchecked. So beware this sleight of hand.

Sound Good? Not so fast: Take a Closer Look at These Terms

- **Natural or All Natural.** *Natural* just means that *some* ingredients are derived from nature. But that doesn't preclude the presence of some highly unnatural additives and hormones.
- **Certified Organic.** The green and white USDA Organic seal means the product was grown/raised, handled, and processed according to certain guidelines—namely, without conventional pesticides or herbicides, synthetic fertilizers, antibiotics, growth hormones, genetic engineering, or irradiation—and produced with an emphasis on soil and water conservation. The term *100% Organic* may be used only on products that contain *only* organic ingredients; *organic* means the product contains at least 95 percent organic ingredients; and *made with organic ingredients* can be found on products containing at least 70 percent organic ingredients. However, a product with less than 70 percent organic content can still claim *Organic ingredients*, but only on the side panel. (You'll read more on this designation in Step #2.)
- **Free Range** *or* **Free-roaming.** Currently these terms are not standardized. You can trust the animal had outdoor access for *some* period each day—but it may have been for just minutes.
- **Low-Fat.** Only foods that contain three grams or less per serving can be labeled low in fat. Eat more than one serving, of course, and it's no longer so low in fat.
- **Whole-Grain** *and* **Multigrain.** Bread, cereal, or cracker labels may tout whole or multigrains regardless of whether they've been processed and stripped of most fiber and nutritional value. *100% whole grain* means it contains no refined flour (a good thing); *made with whole grain* may have a lot or almost no whole grains.
- **Made with Real Fruit.** Are these products made with lots of actual fruit or just drops of fruit juice? There's no way to know.
- **Low Sodium.** Products labeled low in sodium must be 25 percent less salty than the original—but if the food was high in sodium to begin with (e.g., many soups), then you may still get loads of salt.

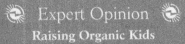

⚙ Expert Opinion ⚙
Raising Organic Kids

By Nell Newman, cofounder of Newman's Own Organics, and author of
The Newman's Own Organics Guide to a Good Life

I don't have kids. I only have chickens. But I do have nephews, and I've seen how tough it can be to get them to eat well. One of them likes only white foods. I hear that's not so rare these days. My mother always says, "I don't remember you kids being so difficult." In our house, the rule was you had to try it. So we tried everything on our plate, even just a bite, or sat there at the table until it got cold. And *then* had to try it.

I think it all comes down to how you start kids off, so it becomes ingrained. To me, the important thing is to give kids an experience of where food comes from. When I was little, I was intrigued by the growing process. I liked gardening; I liked putting that tiny seed in the ground and seeing something come out of it. My mom taught me to cook at an early age, and we used to make pies from the fruit trees that grew in our yard, and omelets from the eggs laid by our chickens. My dad was always picky about his produce. There was a farm stand in Westport, Connecticut, called Rippy's. That's where I learned how to pick a ripe watermelon and what good corn looked like. I was part of the process. We fished in the Long Island Sound and in the river in the backyard for sunnies and trout. We had a great time, and it taught me where food came from. Somebody once asked me, "How did you learn how to clean fish?" I said that one day Dad had to go somewhere and said, "Here, cut it like this and take the guts out." (Mom wouldn't touch it.) Food was a hands-on experience. As a child that was interesting to me.

My nephews live in the house I grew up in but they're much more oriented toward the computer. I told them I didn't want to do the Easter egg hunt on the Internet with kids from all over the world. They didn't get that. They're more removed from nature. I've dragged them out fishing, which they ended up liking even though at first they didn't want to go. When I cooked the fish we caught, I had to make it look like fish sticks. My sister was proud of me for that one.

Kids like to be part of the decision-making process. Next time you go to the store, have them help you read the labels to see what's in things, answer your questions about what the foods are, and help you find foods with the "certified organic" label. If there's a nearby farmers' market, it's a much more interesting experience than the grocery store. Kids can pick their favorite produce and ask the farmers about how they grew it. Kids love meeting farmers.

Things are different today from when I grew up, and it's a lot harder to get kids who are entrenched in their habits to go outside their comfort zones. But I really believe it's just a matter of exposing them early to where food comes from: a field, not a box; a tree, not a jar; a fish, not a stick.

Step #2. The Big O: Go Organic

Organic produce, no longer just the province of sawdust-carpeted health-food stores but increasingly available at a Supermarket Near You, guarantees better, purer food. But it's typically a bit more expensive. Why, then, go the organic route?

The overriding reason is because organic fruits and vegetables are grown without synthetic pesticides or fertilizers. While there's little data on the health effects of eating conventionally grown produce, the potential impact of pesticides on the developing brain and body is no small worry. Farmers and others who work with pesticides have demonstrably elevated rates of asthma, leukemia, and prostate cancer. And while we've made strides in ridding our food of some of the worst chemicals (like DDT) that have the nasty habit of staying in our bodies for an entire lifetime, some of these are still used abroad and may sneak into our food supply through imported produce.

Furthermore, half of our lifetime exposure to pesticides occurs in the first five years of life. Think of it: Pound for pound, kids consume four to

23
number of
elementary-school
children (100
percent of those
tested) whose urine
revealed the
presence of pesti-
cides at the begin-
ning of a study in
Seattle, Washington.

l
number of those
same children
whose urine
contained any
detectable traces of
pesticides after four
days of eating
organic food.
(Environmental Health
Perspectives, 2005)

five times more fruits, veggies, and milk than adults. They may even ingest much more than that because some little kids are "bingers"—while the average child may drink one glass of apple juice a day, others may drink eight. And so children end up more exposed than any of us would want.

I don't mean to scare you. The goal of course is not to avoid fresh fruits and vegetables. We all need plenty of these to help prevent heart disease, diabetes, and colon and other cancers. But switching to organic food immediately lowers pesticide levels in the body. Pregnant women in particular should try to make organic eating a habit for the sake of their developing child. And feeding an infant organic baby food should be a priority.

If you can't buy organic across the board, at least do it for those fruits and vegetables with the highest pesticide levels, known as "The Dirty Dozen." Doing so will right away reduce your family's pesticide exposure by up to 90 percent, according to the Environmental Working Group's investigation. Those on a budget (and who isn't?) should take a look at which produce is the *safest* to buy conventionally.

Is organic more nutritious? Perhaps slightly, though research is preliminary. Some types of organic produce have been found to carry higher levels of vitamin C and other protective antioxidants. But that's not the most compelling reason to eat organic. Next to the health of your kids, perhaps the greatest good is found in supporting farms that grow food in ways that are more protective of nature. Organic farmers generally use less energy, generate less waste, cause less soil erosion, sustain more diversity, enable wildlife to thrive, and provide healthier conditions for workers. Given the growing demands on our land and

---

✂ Copy and Carry ✂
Shopper's Guide to Pesticides in Produce

The Dirty Dozen	The Cleanest 12
Buy These Organic	*Lowest in Pesticides*
Peaches	Onions
Apples	Avocadoes
Sweet bell peppers	Sweet corn (frozen)
Celery	Pineapples
Nectarines	Mangoes
Strawberries	Sweet peas (frozen)
Cherries	Asparagus
Lettuce	Kiwis
Grapes (imported)	Bananas
Pears	Cabbage
Spinach	Broccoli
Potatoes	Eggplant

WORST ⟵ / ⟶ **BEST**

Source: Environmental Working Group, foodnews.org.

---

resources, buying organic is one of the most unambiguously beneficial contributions we can make to the dinner table of the future.

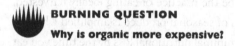

BURNING QUESTION
Why is organic more expensive?

The question might well be rephrased: *Is organic more expensive?"* Because in the long run, it's not.

Regular produce is typically sold at an artificially low price because conventional industrial farming is heavily subsidized by the government. As a result, the s mall and midsize farmer has been put out of business at an alarming rate. From 1993 to 1997, for example, an average of fifty midsize family farms went under *every day*. Giant farms, which benefit most from economies of scale, subsidies, and tax breaks, yield food that's relatively cheap. They also yield a far less diverse range of crops.

Organic farming, on the other hand, which is far more labor-intensive, gets very little say, if any, in federal subsidies. Also, organic farmers can't spray herbicides to get rid of weeds; they do it by hand. Hard labor costs money, and so does certification saying that you don't spray chemicals. So, in fact, the retail price of organic food far more accurately reflects the true cost of growing food right.

Besides, don't forget the massive hidden costs we all pay for conventional farming practices, from contaminated drinking water to soil depletion, and most important, to our health.

 HEALTHY BYTE
Are You a Good Peach or a Bad Peach?

With produce there's a way to tell what you've got: the PLU code on the sticker. Conventionally grown produce carries a four-digit code (e.g., 3577) while organic has five digits beginning with 9 (e.g., 93577). Soon you might find GMO produce beginning with 8 (e.g., 83577), but this labeling is voluntary for producers. The best way to avoid GMO foods is to choose organic when possible.

Step #3. Be a Locavore

Foodies use this term to describe the practice of eating locally harvested, seasonal produce. The freshness of seasonal produce is amplified when it's also local, since it has endured minimal nutritional loss by the time you eat it. Food from local farms is also less likely to have been treated with postharvest pesticides. While it's nearly impossible to identify the pesticides used and the route to transport, say, a bunch of grapes from Chile to your nearest supermarket, foods grown locally afford us a greater sense of control over what we're putting into our bodies. Local food generally uses less packaging, comes in more varieties, and, quite frankly, tastes amazing. We sometimes forget the knee-buckling delight that we get from fresh-picked blueberries or melons or corn. Eat the Seasons (eattheseasons.com) shows which foods are in season each week, the health benefits of those foods, and how long they'll be available. As the saying goes, "Know your farmer, know your food."

DIY

Oh, Pioneer! Freezing Summer Fruit for Winter

Gone is the era when families spent days madly canning freshly harvested berries, peaches, melons, and other summer fruit for the long—and vitamin-deprived—winter. While traditionalists can still play homesteader (you can buy the gold-standard Ball canning kit online), you can also just employ your freezer. Wash, dry, and puree your favorite summer fruits—apricots, nectarines, melons, you name it—scoop them into reusable containers (fill them to the top to avoid freezer burn), label them, and pop them in the freezer. Berries don't even need to be pureed. Enjoy as a topping on yogurt, desserts, or blended into smoothies.

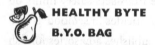

HEALTHY BYTE
B.Y.O. BAG

The average American family of four tosses out about fifteen hundred plastic bags a year; each one takes up to one thousand years to decompose. Skip the moral dilemma and bring a reusable bag—organic canvas, cloth, nylon—to the store. If mesh bags are too tree-huggery, bring a tote: one of those giant Lands' End monogrammed canvas bags, or a chic Louis Vuitton tote (well, maybe not for leaky groceries). Some stores, like Whole Foods, will reward you for it with a small discount.

Step #4. Fish for a Cleaner Catch

There are many reasons to hook your family on fish: The omega-3 acids in fatty fish, especially sardines, mackerel, and wild salmon, spur fetal

and baby brain growth. Most seafood is high in protein and low in unhealthy fats, so it makes a great alternative to red meat. For adults, the
nutrients in fish and other seafood help to prevent heart attacks by lowering the bad cholesterol (LDL) and raising the good kind (HDL).

But you've no doubt heard that eating seafood has its risks, mainly from
industrial chemicals and other pollutants that build up in the fish we eat.
Two common pollutants—mercury and PCBs—are linked to learning and
memory problems in children, thyroid problems, and possibly cancer. Because they alter normal brain development, these chemicals have the greatest impact on babies and children. Both mercury and PCBs accumulate in
the body over time: PCBs are removed from the body very slowly (it takes
about ten years to get rid of half of last night's dinner); mercury has a half-
life of seventy days (so a woman who hopes to become pregnant can clear
her body in about one year). These substances can also pass from a pregnant woman or a nursing mother to her baby. So it's especially important
for children, teenage girls, and women who are pregnant, trying to conceive, or nursing to avoid fish that are high in mercury or PCBs.

When you're fishing for answers on what seafood is okay to eat and
how much, what's the best guide to use? The FDA sets safety limits on
concentrations of mercury and a number of pesticides in seafood as well
as arsenic in shellfish. The EPA, meanwhile, publishes advisories for fish
caught in specific bodies of water. These agencies don't always agree on
what's safe, though. For example, the FDA says it's okay to ingest higher
levels of mercury than the EPA does.

Don't let all this talk of awful chemicals make you fishphobic. In most
cases the health benefits of eating seafood outweigh the risks as long as
you make smart choices. How to do this? Know your fish. I keep a fish
chart in my wallet that I like to whip out in restaurants. (It also lists the
most overfished species so I can eat seafood knowing I'm not contributing to the end of biodiversity.) I'll give you that list in a moment, but first,
a few rules of thumb:

Let the big one get away. The bigger (and more predatory) the fish, the
higher the mercury, dioxin, and PCB contamination, so skip the shark,

swordfish, king mackerel, tilefish (from the Gulf of Mexico), and big-eye ahi tuna. These types tend to accumulate high concentrations of contaminants because they eat lots of other tainted fish over a long life span. Much better for you: the little guys, like anchovies, sardines, and cod.

Be wary of bottom feeders. Pollutants tend to settle on the bottom of waterways, where lobsters, mollusks, and their pals lurk. Toxic substances are unlikely to be washed away or, due to lack of sunlight, to biodegrade.

Tune in to your tuna habit. The most recent government data show that, on average, canned white albacore tuna has three times more mercury than canned chunk light tuna, sometimes exceeding the government specified limit. Children, teen girls, pregnant women (or those trying to conceive) and nursing mothers, and even men trying to become parents, should avoid white albacore tuna or tuna steaks. The EPA advises that pregnant women can safely have up to twelve ounces of chunk light tuna per week. Different opinions making you crazy? Use the Environmental Working Group's tuna calculator at ewg.org/tunacalculator to find out how much might be best for you. Keep in mind that you'll want to weigh that number against your total fish consumption.

Go wild. Farmed fish are raised in close quarters and are treated with pesticides and fed antibiotics to minimize lice and disease, a practice that pollutes waterways. Salmon, the third most popular fish in the United States, is particularly problematic when raised this way. Farmed salmon have been shown to have higher concentrations of pollutants—up to ten times more PCBs—than wild.

Though wild is the superior stuff, it can be significantly more expensive than farmed. How to tell whether fish is indeed wild? The Marine Stewardship Council (msc.org) certifies wild Alaska salmon. Otherwise—and for other fish—you'll have to ask your fishmonger or waiter, and trust their response.

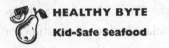

HEALTHY BYTE
Kid-Safe Seafood

Kid Safe Seafood offers clear information about how much fish—and what types—kids can eat, and keeps a database of healthy recipes. See kidsafeseafood.org.

Meanwhile, you can choose alternative sources of omega-3 fatty acids, which are so crucial for brain development, such as walnuts, flax seed, olive oil, and eggs of chicken fed a special diet.

HEALTHY BYTE
One Fish, Two Fish, Best Fish

This checklist from Oceans Alive, part of the Environmental Defense Network, can help you choose fish that are the healthiest for the oceans and safest to eat. The underlined fish varieties are high in omega-3s and low in contaminants. The varieties in *italics* are high in mercury or PCBs.

BEST	WORST
Abalone (U.S. farmed)	*Caviar (wild)*
<u>Anchovies</u>	*Chilean sea bass/Toothfish*
Arctic char (farmed)	*Cod (Atlantic)*
Catfish (U.S. farmed)	*Grouper*
Caviar (U.S. farmed)	*Halibut (Atlantic)*
Clams (farmed)	*Marlin*
Crab (Dungeness, snow, stone)	Monkfish/Goosefish
Crawfish (U.S.)	*Orange roughy*
Halibut (Pacific/Alaska)	*Rockfish/Rock cod (Pacific)*
Herring (<u>Atlantic: U.S., Canada</u>)	Salmon *(Atlantic/farmed)*
Mackerel (<u>Atlantic</u>)	*Shark*
Mahimahi (Atlantic: U.S.)	Shrimp/prawns (imported)
Mussels (farmed)	Skate
<u>Oysters (farmed)</u>	Snapper
<u>Sablefish/Black cod (Alaska)</u>	Sturgeon *(wild)*

Salmon (<u>wild Alaska, canned pink/sockeye</u>)

<u>Sardines</u>

Scallops (bay: farmed)

Shrimp (Canada, Oregon pink, U.S. farmed)

Spot prawns

Striped bass (farmed)

Sturgeon (U.S. farmed)

Tilapia (U.S.)

Swordfish (imported)

Tilefish

Tuna *(bluefin)*

Source: Reprinted with permission from Oceans Alive. For more information see oceansalive.org.

Parentblog
If I Could Do It Again
By Gayle King, magazine editor/TV personality/radio host

When it comes to food, I'm not that green. I never wanted to make my own apple juice or puree my own peas. But now I make healthy choices about food, and I only wish someone had really, *really* explained the consequences of not doing that when you're around young kids. I always heard, *It's important to eat your vegetables.* We all did. But it wasn't until I was older that I realized just how important it is, and what damage can be caused by not appreciating that.

When my kids were younger, if they didn't eat what I put out for them, it was no big deal. I didn't enforce it (and I hate the word *enforcer* because it sounds so punitive). I wasn't a big vegetable eater myself. I never said anything to them like, *These carrots and spinach are so great, I can't wait for you to taste them.* It was just so much less friction to do SpaghettiOs or pizza again. And since I'm not a great cook, it was easier in that way, too.

As my son got older, his habits, like most kids his age, were pretty much set. In high school, we had the three-bite rule: He had to take three bites of spinach or broccoli or whatever. Sure enough, he took his three bites and that was it. There was no pleasure involved whatsoever. For him it was like a prison sentence.

Now my son is in his junior year of college and I have to bribe him to eat a salad. Recently we went out to eat and I said, "Will, you've got to order vegetables." And he replied, "Well, I wasn't taught that." And you know what? He was absolutely right. He wasn't.

Fortunately my kids are very healthy. But I would have handled things differently. It's just about my biggest regret as a parent. I would have made sure to start them by two or three years old. Since they gravitate toward sweets at around that age, I would have made some more deals with them. Instead of letting them eat Ho Hos and Twinkies and saying, *If you're good, I'll let you have some ice cream,* why couldn't I have said, *If you're good, I'm going to let you have an apple?* I would have made a point, when my child was going over to other people's houses, to ask if they wouldn't mind giving him fruit or veggies for a snack. I'm not saying that, if I had it to do again, my son would never have gone to one of those ice cream birthday parties. But I think I could have incorporated these situations into our lives better. I would have said, *Look, if we're going to eat this ice cream or dessert or whatever, then let's skip it next week.* I would have started cooking with canola oil instead of corn oil a lot sooner.

It's about education and moderation. For instance, fried foods: There are ways to get the taste of fried chicken without actually frying it. Same with potatoes: You oven-bake them and get the same flavor without putting them in all that grease and oil.

Both my children are in college now and I've come to see how important it is to start your kids early on healthy foods, and to treat those foods as if they really taste good, whether you think so or not. After all, they pick up their cues from you. Kids learn manners from parents, they learn hatreds and prejudices from them, why shouldn't they learn from them the beauty of an asparagus? One mother said to me, *Yes, I did that and they still don't like veggies.* I guess you need to do it in a way that doesn't force them, that celebrates what is good about healthy foods, and do it in small doses.

Everybody wants to raise happy, healthy, well-adjusted children—emphasis on that word *healthy*. Like I said, I'm not one of those mothers who could ever have grown her own garden, but if I had to do it all over again, I would really celebrate the joys of carrots and broccoli and spinach. I certainly would have felt better had I tried. And, of course, my children would have, too.

Step #5. Junk It: Sidestep the Worst Preservatives and Additives

I thought I'd seen it all when I was cruising the yogurt section of my supermarket and spotted blue, cotton-candy flavored yogurt for kids. Manufacturers are all too aware that children are compulsively drawn to Technicolor foods and those that are sweet or salty. Since getting kids to eat well is an exercise in triage as you figure the pros and cons of cost, time, and availability, you might be tempted to take the path of least resistance: chicken nuggets, flame-colored mac 'n' cheese, blue yogurt. That's fine sometimes. But the chemical additives—preservatives, flavors, and colors—found in these types of food have a disproportionately greater health impact on children than on adults.

Food additives are largely present in nonorganic processed and packaged foods. To keep most additives out of your child's diet, serving fresh produce, organic protein sources, whole grain, and USDA organic-packaged foods are a great start. Besides, you can always make healthy versions of your brood's favorites. For homemade nuggets, just dip chicken tenders into yogurt and crushed cereal and bake at 400°F for about twenty minutes; or make a cheesier version of macaroni and cheese using real cheddar or Emmental.

Kids are going to eat their share of junk, so play detective and sleuth out the unhealthiest additives. Bonus points if you can get them to help you spot some of the following ingredients on labels. (For a complete list of food additives to avoid, see the Center for Science in the Public Interest's site: cspinet.org/reports/chemcuisine.htm.)

Pick "preservative-free." Preservatives help extend the shelf (or refrigerator) life of food, but their ingredients are often unsafe. For instance, butylated hydroxyanisole (BHA), which keeps oils from going rancid, is listed as a probable human carcinogen by the Department of Health and Human Services (remarkably, the FDA says it's okay to eat it). The other biggie in this category to look for on labels—and to avoid—is BHT, or butylated hydroxytoluene.

Don't get sweet on sugar substitutes. Kids scarf down way too much sugar, but artificial sweeteners shouldn't be a compromise. Aspartame (known as NutraSweet and Equal), found in diet sodas and in some kids' products like vitamins and toothpaste, and saccharine (Sweet'n Low) each have a history of controversy. Though no negative health effects have been proven definitively in humans, many scientists have suggested a correlation between these faux sugars and consequences from headaches to cancer. As for sucralose (Splenda), there hasn't been adequate research to draw conclusions. Stevia, a natural sweetener made from an herb, is a relatively new sweetener that appears to be safer than the others. The bottom line: Kids should eat less sugar, and less fake sugar.

Low-dose your high-fructose corn syrup. This sweetener, made from processed corn syrup and used in everything from breads and cereals to soft drinks and salad dressings, is common in food because it's sweeter and a whole lot cheaper than cane sugar. Many experts blame it for contributing to the rise in childhood obesity. Animal studies have linked high-fructose corn syrup to diabetes and high cholesterol, though it's unclear whether the same is true in humans. The fact is, we consume too much high-fructose corn syrup in foods that carry little or no nutritional value. Read labels: If it's listed among the first couple of ingredients, put the product back on the shelf.

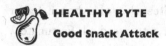

HEALTHY BYTE
Good Snack Attack

Kids should try to snack from two different food groups, twice a day, to be sure to get an adequate range of nutrients, according to Nicole Meadow, M.P.N., R.D., and founder of NutritionWise. Some of her favorite kid-approved noshes:

Yogurt (6-ounce container, low-fat) and fruit

Nuts (1/4 cup) and dried fruit (preservative-free)

1/2 Whole-grain pita with scrambled eggs and veggies

Carrots and hummus

Ants on a log (celery with peanut butter or cream cheese and raisins)

Whole-grain pita (baked in the oven into chips) with hummus

Smoothie (milk or soy milk with 1/2 banana and frozen fruit—strawberries, blueberries, mangoes)

Hard-boiled egg and a slice of whole-grain toast

Apple or banana with peanut butter (1 tablespoon)

Whole-grain crackers with cheese

Fruit and string cheese

Avocado (1/4 cup) and whole-grain crackers

Yogurt with 1/4 cup low-fat granola

Fruit and cheese kabobs

Turkey breast slices, and/or rolled low-fat cheese slices and sliced pear, apple, or peaches

1/2 Grilled cheese sandwich (with thin slices of tomato) on thin sliced whole-wheat bread

Cut out trans fats. Found in cookies, crackers, icing, chips, french fries, doughnuts, microwave popcorn, and many other snack and fried foods, trans fats—known also as partially hydrogenated oils—are artificial fats that make oil more solid and thereby increase a product's shelf life. They're the most harmful fat in the food supply, contributing to heart disease and high cholesterol levels. Kids fed diets high in fast food, stick margarine, and factory-made baked goods runs a higher risk for heart disease than kids who eat healthier foods.

What should you look for on the label? Steer clear of hydrogenated or partially hydrogenated canola, soybean, or cottonseed oil. Fortunately, some companies have eliminated trans fats, particularly in products targeted to kids. A couple of fast-food chains have done the same, and trans fats are considered such artery cloggers that New York City voted to ban the ingredient from all food sold in restaurants—the first such measure in the nation.

Color them naturally. Conjure those blue yogurts, neon-colored fruit drinks, and snacks: You don't need to read the label to know these artificial colors can't be good for your kids. In particular, avoid FD&C blues #1 and 2; green #3; and yellows #5 and 6.

Sodium nitrites. Used to preserve cured and processed meats—bacon, sausage, ham—and to keep them looking red and juicy, these compounds have been linked to various types of cancer in lab tests. Cured meat shouldn't be a daily staple of your kids' lunch boxes. This goes for pregnant women, too. Fortunately, nitrite-free meats are getting easier to find.

Say N-O to MSG. Monosodium glutamate is a flavor enhancer found principally in soups, salad dressings, chips, shake-on seasonings, and fast-food Asian cuisine; its taste is so potent that it allows companies to use fewer real food ingredients (like the chicken in chicken soup). Studies have shown that some people are sensitive to MSG, with reactions ranging from headache and shortness of breath to changes in heart rate (these occur because MSG directly attacks neurons, and at high doses can even kill nerve cells). Note that hydrolized protein, a flavoring added to some canned and prepared foods, contains MSG, but MSG isn't required to appear on the label.

Cut out caffeine. Kids typically encounter caffeine in iced tea and colas (chocolate- and coffee-flavored yogurts contain a bit of naturally occurring caffeine, too), and teens have likely already gotten swept up in the double-macchiato/high-octane latte craze. You want to minimize their caffeine exposure for two main reasons: (1) it's a stimulant and kids are energetic enough without it; and (2) it's mildly addictive, so you don't want your child experiencing the groaning lethargy of withdrawal.

Parentblog
That's Your Intuition Talking
By Gigi Lee Chang, founder of Plum Organics

Every morning for practically my entire life, my mother has religiously made a shake of fruits and vegetables. I grew up in California, so whatever she had in the house—cucumbers, tomatoes, melon, peaches—she would blend up. Then she added milk (it sounds good up to there, but that's where she loses me). She claims it's a great way to get all your vitamins and fiber in one glass. When she's done she puts the leftovers on her face. She says, "You're buying all those alpha-whatevers, and this is the most natural way to get antioxidants on your skin." Her youthful complexion is proof that it works.

So maybe it's no surprise that I got into the organic baby food business—though I certainly didn't plan to. Once my son, Cato, was old enough to eat solids, my Kidco food mill was my favorite accessory. I'd grind up everything, even leftover Chinese food, and he'd eat it all. It's not that I thought the jarred food was bad; I just thought I could do it better. I don't have a nutrition degree; it's simply that my husband and I like to cook (an oddity in New York City). I figured if I had the major food groups covered and fed him a range of colors, he'd probably be okay. The downside was that I was working full-time in advertising and spending one of every three weekends making the stuff and freezing it. But Cato ate everything I put in front of him, so on another level it was easy.

That same maternal instinct that inspired me to make baby food has helped me navigate many of the confusing choices of new parenthood. For example, during the first week of my son's life, I looked in his diaper and saw all these little gel crystals from the moisture. I thought, *Yuck, I don't know what these are, but I don't want them next to my son's skin, so I* switched to eco-friendly diapers. Or when I washed his clothes in traditional detergent, thinking you had to use it for babies, it smelled so strong and was so brightly colored, it didn't seem right. Now I use the nonchemical laundry detergent. (I'm sure you've had these revelations, too; all I can say is go with your gut.) I've never considered myself very granola, but maybe I'm crunchier than I thought.

That instinct also gave me the confidence to leave my job in advertising to start Plum Organics. I know so many women who want to make healthier food choices for their kids but don't have the time or confidence in the kitchen. This was a way I could help. When I started researching my business, I found data showing that taste preferences are formed by age two. I believe it, because today, at four, my son eats everything—literally.

Below is the recipe for one of our most popular dishes. I'd give you the recipe for Cato's favorite ever—chicken livers with rutabaga—but I'm not sure you'd want that!

Plum Organics Super Greens Baby Food

Makes approximately 6 portions

½ cup baby spinach leaves*
½ cup green beans
1 cup frozen sweet peas

Boil a pot of water.
Blanch the spinach for 1 minute. Steam the green beans until tender and cooked through. Soak the frozen peas in a bowl of hot water for 5 minutes.

Puree all ingredients in a food processor for 2–3 minutes until desired consistency (adding a little water if smoother texture is desired).

*You can also use frozen baby spinach leaves. If using frozen, soak leaves in hot water for 2 minutes instead of blanching.

Keep an eye out for GMOs. Genetically modified or engineered food (GMO or GE) is a way for farmers to create heartier, pest-resistant crops—for instance, by breeding a pesticide right into the grain—and so far is limited principally to canola, soybean, and corn. GMO foods are commonly used for animal feed, but have entered our lives quietly in the form of additives to packaged food. We don't have an exact figure for how pervasive GMO processed foods are, but roughly 60 percent of processed food in U.S. grocery stores contain at least one soybean product, and more than half of our soybean crops are genetically modified.

There are no long-term health safety tests or labeling for these foods. U.S. government regulators and biotech companies say GMO foods are safe, but they're banned throughout Europe. Some research shows a worrisome impact on plants and wildlife, and that food allergens may be transmitted through bioengineering, according to the watchdog group Beyond Pesticides.

In the meantime, if your child is prone to food allergies, give her natural and GMO-free (some labels will tout it) snack alternatives, such as fresh fruits and vegetables, nuts, cheese, and yogurt—which may even be a sound policy for the nonallergic.

Parentblog
Yes, Kids Can Get Hooked On Health Food
By Gwyneth Paltrow, actress

My mom has always been conscious of the environment and health issues. When I was growing up, we would go to farmers' markets and even had wheatgrass in the kitchen. She started a curbside recycling program in Santa Monica in the 1970s, and each week I drove with her to the recycling center. She says I used to roll down the window to yell, "You're polluting!" at truck drivers in their semis. I was three years old.

It wasn't until later that I understood the harm that can come from pesticides and other chemicals in foods. As soon as I did, I tried to eat organic, locally, and foods that weren't processed or full of preservatives. That was reinforced when I became a parent. When I would read about what pesticides do to insects and small animals, I thought, Why would I expose my child to that? It didn't make sense.

From the beginning, my kids have eaten organic. I make a lot of their foods myself. Some people say it sounds difficult—or crazy—but I never found it so. When I'd go to the health-food store and see organic baby food in a jar that had been sitting on a shelf for six or nine months, I thought, How good can *that* be? So I didn't find it tough to make my own. It's much tougher for me to open a jar that's been sitting on a shelf for God knows how long and then feed it to my child.

Once Apple and then Moses were old enough to eat solids, I would make a big batch of organic brown rice and keep it in the fridge for a couple of days. I'd puree it with organic vegetables that I'd steamed. It's easy to make organic oats for them in the morning with a little pure maple syrup (it breaks down slowly so there's no "insulin bombing," the way there is with sugar), or full-fat live yogurt with flax meal and fruit puree. Since we don't eat red meat, we cook a lot of bean and whole-grain combos for a complete protein. Once you've made your own baby food, it's easy to keep up as the kids get older: brown rice and black beans with soft tortillas and guacamole—they love dipping. Little sandwiches of whole-grain mini pitas with hummus.

Food was the beginning of my awareness of the toxic substances we ingest. Now we've done other things to protect our family's health, from installing a water filtration system to sleeping on organic mattresses and using nontoxic shampoos. I try to open the windows in the day—an old-fashioned airing out—even in winter, because the air inside the house is often more polluted than the air outside. I read a lot—moms e-mail each other links to studies and health alerts, the kind that keep you up at night. But I try not to get hysterical about it. I'm not doing all this to turn my kids into freaks—I just want them to be as healthy as they possibly can. I don't want to fill them with anxiety. I keep the anxiety part to myself.

An ancient Chinese proverb says something like, "Food and medicine have the same root." The more I learn about food, the more amazed I am at how their properties can basically fix anything. My main feeling, honestly: The purer you keep your body, the healthier you will be. Of course there will be toxic chemicals, hormones, and heavy metals that come into your and your kids' lives and nostrils and mouths. But I believe that eating well is the best start for living well.

Moses's Brown Rice Baby Food

Brown rice is naturally sweet and babies love it. As Moses got bigger, I made the puree coarser. It can last in the fridge for a couple of days.

Puree 1 cup cooked brown rice with 1½ cups unsweetened rice milk (adjust amounts for consistency). Steam any of your child's favorite veggies—sweet potatoes, peas, broccoli—and puree that, too. Mix the purees in whatever amounts your kid likes.

Apple's Organic Roast Veggie Sticks

My kids eat these with their fingers. When they cool, the sticks are all caramelized and delicious.

Peel carrots, sweet potatoes, and parsnips and cut into thick french fry–size pieces. Toss with a drizzling of olive oil and a bit of salt and pepper, and roast for 30 minutes at 400°F. After 20 minutes, remove from the oven, stir in some maple syrup, then return to the oven until lightly browned.

Step #6. A Livelier Stock: Organic Beef and Dairy

Note to carnivores: Organic meat eliminates your exposure to the hormones animals are fed to bulk them up faster, the antibiotics they've been given to fight infection, and the pesticides they're exposed to in their feed. Extra hormones in a child's diet may affect growth and interfere with natural maturation patterns. There's no solid proof that hormone-dosed beef is a health risk to adults, but there's no evidence to the contrary, either. Ninety percent of American feedlot cattle is injected with growth hormones—that's why Europe and Canada won't import it. (If you see the label NO HORMONES ADMINISTERED on pork or poultry products, don't be impressed: The USDA bans the use of hormones on these meats.)

If your child eats beef, there's also value in keeping it as lean as possible. Traces of dioxin concentrate in animal fat (including farm-raised fish). The less fat, the less dioxin exposure.

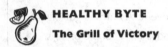

HEALTHY BYTE
The Grill of Victory

Try not to overcook your 'cue: Charred meat can contain polycyclic aromatic hydrocarbons (PAHs) and heterocyclic amines (HCAs), which can increase the risk of some cancers, according to the National Cancer Institute. Use less fatty meats, which don't drip as much onto the coals, causing smoke flare-ups (PAHs form in the smoke and are then deposited on the meat). Put a layer of foil between meat and coals and cook at lower temperatures (which reduces the formation of HCAs). Then again, you don't want to undercook meat, either, or you heighten the risk of salmonella and E. coli.

Got organic milk? It costs a bit more than regular milk but the health benefits are worth it. As with meat, organic dairy products come from animals raised without synthetic interference. To boost conventional milk production, dairy farmers inject their herd with recombinant bovine growth hormones or rBGH, which tricks their bodies into making more milk (read about the downside of rBGH in the box on the next page). Also, these cows are frequently given antibiotics to keep them from spreading disease.

Kids drink lots of milk, so switch to organic—and organic versions of other dairy products like cheese and yogurt. If milk doesn't contain growth hormones, the carton will usually say so. Smaller dairies tend not to use hormones because of the expense and the harm to cows: another good reason to buy from local, smaller suppliers.

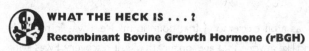

WHAT THE HECK IS . . . ?
Recombinant Bovine Growth Hormone (rBGH)

Since its approval by the FDA in 1994, rBGH has been used to boost cows' milk output by as much as 25 percent. The drug is injected into anywhere from 5 to 30 percent of cows in the United States. Though its manufacturer contends that milk produced with rBGH is no less safe than non-rBGH milk, others disagree: Use of rBGH has been linked to breast and prostate cancers in animals. What's more, the growth factor it produces finds its way into the milk of cows, which, when ingested, can be absorbed into the bloodstream, where it can potentially affect hormones.

Egg-cellence. In recent years, egg consumption took a hit because of fears that it jacked up cholesterol levels. But eggs really are the incredible, edible things the old jingle used to tout: They are super sources of protein, vitamins A, D, B_{12}, B_2, niacin, and folic acid. Organic egg hens roam free and are fed grains without chemicals, hormones, or antibiotics. They may also be more nutritious than regular eggs: A recent survey found that eggs from free-range hens had three times the vitamin E, two times the omega-3 fatty acids, and seven times the beta carotene (a form of vitamin A) of conventional eggs, while averaging one-third the cholesterol.

Parentblog
The Good Enough Environmentalist
By Carolyn Murphy, model, actress, activist

One day back in 1995, I was traveling for a modeling job and browsing a row of magazines in the airport. The cover of *Time* caught my eye: It showed an overblown tomato and a headline about genetically modified foods. The idea that scientists didn't know the health consequences of these manipulated foods really horrified me, especially having grown up in Florida, where produce is so abundant and fresh. I decided to start educating myself on the topic.

Now, I was a bit extreme at that point in my life. I was in my early twenties, and like anyone that age, on a path of self-discovery. I was living in Manhattan's meatpacking district and went completely vegetarian—how could I not with all that bloody beef hanging in my doorway? I would only shop at health-food stores. I was disgusted that the FDA didn't force companies that made, grew, or distributed food to tell us what was in it. I started speaking out about it to educators, breaking down the "true cost" and price differences of organic for economically disadvantaged kids and families who couldn't afford the more expensive stuff. I was obsessed with figuring out a way to make healthy food available for everyone. I was discovering things and getting excited about them, but I went a little radical.

Then reality set in. As I got older, and especially after I had my daughter, Dylan, in 2000, I realized I couldn't manage every single thing. It was hard enough to maintain my own household and, most important, to be a good mother. I'm traveling, rushing through the airport, and there I am, eating french fries—and you know what? I'm not going to throw them out because they were cooked in lard instead of olive oil. Part of the challenge of living a healthy life is knowing what to be wary of, but it's also knowing when and how to be realistic. After that foray in my twenties, I've opted not to get on a soapbox. In my home, though, I do what I can—choosing only certain toys for my daughter, purifying my water, using nontoxic cleaning products, and finishing my floors naturally. I've carried my own reusable grocery bags for years. To me, being a realist doesn't mean giving in but starting small, writing out a list, and naming your top priority (mine was eating healthy). From there, you branch out.

I do have a philosophy about all this: Living in a more healthful way takes education, integration, and discipline. Education, because you have to inform yourself about the facts and the options—sorting through articles on Google or reading relevant books. Integration, because you have to live in the world; you can't lock yourself away on an organic farm (though sometimes I fantasize about it). Discipline, be-

> cause it's so easy to give in to the temptations of our disposable cul-
> ture. And finally, there's also modification, because over the years you
> have to adjust how you do things, depending on how far you're willing
> to go and what you're capable of.
>
> Okay, maybe I do have a little bit of the radical in me still.

Step #7. Be Alert to Food Allergies

It's likely that when you were growing up you didn't know any kids with
severe food allergies—or if you did, they were sort of a classroom curiosity. Now, of course, schools across the country have instituted peanut-
free zones, and airlines have replaced their little bags of nuts with
pretzels. Approximately 12 million Americans now suffer from food allergies, including anywhere from 5 to 7.5 percent of children; between
1997 and 2002 the number of children under five with peanut allergies
doubled, according to the CDC. For some, allergies are an extreme lifestyle inconvenience; for a small minority, they can be deadly.

Any food can cause an allergic reaction, but 90 percent of all food allergies are caused by one of the following: wheat, eggs, milk, peanuts,
tree nuts, soy, fish, and shellfish. An allergic reaction is how the immune
system responds to a substance that the body mistakes as harmful.
When the body becomes "sensitized" to an allergenic food, it creates
antibodies to fight it off. These antibodies release a cascade of chemicals, including histamines, to protect the body, but these immune chemicals can also harm the respiratory and cardiovascular systems, skin, and
the gastrointestinal tract.

What's causing this allergy increase among kids isn't well understood. However, one prevailing theory, known as the "hygiene hypothesis," postulates that we're *too* clean, thanks to cleansers like
antibacterial soaps, which leave the body with few "real" bacterial in-
vaders to attack, thus the body instead overreacts to very low threats,
like nut proteins.

Watch for symptoms. Physical reactions to food allergies can range from mouth tingling, swelling of the tongue and throat, difficulty breathing, and hives to vomiting, abdominal cramps, diarrhea, drop in blood pressure, and loss of consciousness, according to foodallergy.org. Symptoms can appear within minutes to two hours after ingestion. If you observe *any* of these, call your pediatrician. He or she will then likely perform a RAST (RadioAllergoSorbent Test) to look for antibodies in blood.

3.1 million number of school-age children with food allergies. (The Food Allergy and Anaphylaxis Network, 2007)

Fortunately, most people outgrow their food allergies, though peanut, fish, and shellfish allergies are often considered lifelong. They may become so severe that a pediatrician may have to resort to medicines like antihistamines and epinephrine to prevent a serious or even deadly reaction.

Know what your kids are eating. If allergies run in your family, be careful when introducing new foods to your baby or toddler. Processed foods are likely to contain traces of peanut, soy, and other allergens, so read the labels carefully. If in doubt about a food that your child really wants, call the manufacturer to make sure it doesn't contain an ingredient that could make your child sick.

Alert your school and other parents. Talk to the principal, your child's teachers, the school nurse, and also the parents of the other kids in the classroom to tip them off about your child's allergy. You'll need to stay on top of the snacks served at school, and have an emergency plan in place. For free downloadable letters to parents, teachers, and principals, or to order a set of "Allergy Kids" stickers for lunch boxes to warn caregivers of specific allergies, visit allergykids .com. Some other useful sites: foodallergy.org, aaaai.org, and statkids.com.

Parentblog
Sometimes It Takes a Mom
By Robyn O'Brien, founder of Allergy Kids

I had four kids in five years. It's so crazy-busy around our house, it's enough of a challenge just getting everyone to eat something at all. For breakfast one morning last year, when my youngest child was nine months old, I made scrambled eggs for all the kids. But my baby, Tory, didn't really seem to want them; she was fussing in her high chair and pushing away the eggs so I figured she was tired and put her down for a nap. A few minutes later, I went to check on her, looked down in the crib—and her whole face was swollen. I turned to my older three and asked accusingly, "What did you guys *do?*" But they just gave me those blank little kid stares in return. And that's when I got really scared.

Now, I'm from Houston, which was not a particularly healthy place—I certainly ate my share of Twinkies and po' boys, and putting three square meals on the table was pretty much all my mother worried about when it came to food. So I was completely clueless about food allergies, which is what my pediatrician diagnosed when I called him. And that's when my education began. That night I sat down at the computer and started researching, and I was stunned at how prevalent the problem had become in the last ten years and how little information there really was about it. I thought, it's tough enough to protect my child in my own home; how will I protect her when she's old enough to be at school? Or at friends' houses? It dawned on me that there had to be a universal symbol for food allergies the way there's a pink ribbon for breast cancer, so allergy kids could be identified. And so that night I sat down and sketched out that symbol, which became the bright green "stop sign" shape stickers I've been trying to get into the hands of parents of the millions of children with allergies.

As I researched my questions about food allergies (*Exactly what changed that peanut allergies have doubled between 1997 and 2002? What's different about our food that suddenly in the last ten years peanut butter and jelly sandwiches are like ticking bombs at the lunchroom table? What connection might chemical additives in foods, which are banned in*

Europe, where the allergy rate is lower than here, have to do with all this?) I discovered that the junk-food industry underwrites a lot of the research. Hmm…pretty interesting. I love research; I was an equity analyst on a hedge fund for years. And so my husband basically lost me for months as I went completely under—digging through previously undisclosed studies, looking for answers. I'm still working on it, along with many concerned scientists and activists who are homing in on new explanations.

This whole journey has taken me to a place I never imagined I'd be. I've met so many smart people—farmers, scientists, researchers, activists. I just have to pinch myself. Sometimes it just takes a passionate mom. We all have her in us.

Step #8: Get Prep Schooled

Maybe you've brought into your home the healthiest foods you could find. There still may be unseen enemies to vanquish—microscopic interlopers like bacteria that can make you sick.

Wash your hands. Hands are major culprits in spreading bacteria. Wash with soap and water before and after handling foods, especially meat and poultry.

Clean your produce. Don't bother with expensive spray solutions. Just give a quick cold rinse to all fruits and vegetables (even organic—about one in four bears some pesticide residue, usually as a result of "pesticide drift"). For firm-skinned food, use a gentle scrub brush; if leafy or soft (lettuce, spinach, broccoli, strawberries), soak for a minute and separate leaves or parts. You're removing some pesticide residue and other chemicals, as well as microorganisms such as E. coli, which may have climbed aboard your spinach between the picking and your pot. True, these days lots of produce is pre-washed before it's packaged, and I admit

ENERGY SAVER
Cut your cooking time
Saving time is always a plus, but how about saving energy in the kitchen, too? Defrost in the fridge instead of the microwave. Use the window on your oven instead of opening the door to peek at food. Cook double portions, so next time you only need to reheat.

I sometimes eat it straight from the bag. But it's a worthwhile precaution to rinse again. To be extra careful, make up a produce wash of one part white vinegar to four parts water and keep it in a spray bottle by the sink to deep-six any microbes. Also, peel fruits and vegetables when you can and discard the outer leaves of leafy veggies.

Mind your meat. Raw meat and poultry may carry microbes like salmonella or E. coli. If you put meat down on a counter or other surface, clean it up. But, as explained in the previous chapter, you don't need an antibacterial cleanser; these contain triclosan, which is good neither for you nor the environment. Scrubbing with regular soap and warm water suffices. Never put anything on a plate that previously held raw meat (a common mistake of the addled barbecuer). And once again, wash your hands after handling it.

Keep cutting boards clean. You need at least two of these: one for meat, one for everything else. There's some debate about whether wood or plastic is preferable, but a thorough scrubbing with warm soapy water makes the issue moot.

Sanitize sponges. These are prime breeding grounds for bacteria, which will be wiped onto every surface of the kitchen if you let your sponges go too long. Microwave them on high for at least a minute to kill microbes, or toss them in the dishwasher. Sea sponges or biodegradable cellulose sponges are eco-friendlier than synthetic ones. When sponges start to crumble, toss them. And don't forget to launder your dish towels regularly; these have a way of hanging around the kitchen until they're stiff with grime.

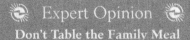

Expert Opinion
Don't Table the Family Meal
By Nicole Meadow, pediatric nutritionist, founder of NutritionWise

With ridiculously busy schedules for everyone, it's easy to understand how the tradition of the family meal has disappeared in so many households. Yet regular mealtime together not only can help strengthen family ties but lead to better health—physical and mental,—in children. A 2004 University of Minnesota study showed a correlation between frequent family meals and better nutritional intake, and decreased risk for unhealthy weight control practices and substance abuse; a 2000 Harvard study asserted that families who ate together every day or almost every day consumed a higher volume of important nutrients and less overall fat than less-frequent family diners. Family mealtime promotes social skills, of course, but it's also fun. While many parents may feel it's too late to (re-)institute family mealtime, including the kids in the process can work wonders:

Start small. Aim for a family meal once a week. When you achieve that, go for more.

Include the kids in the preparation. Have them help plan the night's (or week's) menu, shop for groceries, cook, or set the table.

Have one "kids' choice night." Let them pick what everyone eats for dinner.

Start a ritual at mealtimes. When I was growing up, we each had to share "one good and one bad" thing from our day. Come up with your own engaging ritual.

Get them to model positive dining habits. You're showcasing that a meal is a balanced collection of healthful foods, that there's a wide variety of delicious food (don't just tell them to try new foods but try them yourself), that one should eat slowly and display good manners.

Step #9. Toss Your Teflon

So what if you'll never again be able to fry an egg that slides off the pan like an ice cube? PFOA, the chemical used to make Teflon and other nonstick surfaces, is now found in the blood of nearly every American and has been listed by the EPA as a "likely human carcinogen." When nonstick pans reach very high temperatures—and tests prove they do—the coating breaks apart and emits potentially cancerous particles and gases that are linked to eye and respiratory inflammation (it's even been blamed for the deaths of pet birds!). After government pressure, Du-Pont and seven other companies that make PFOA have agreed to eliminate its use by 2015. Don't wait until then; opt for one of the following materials:

Stainless steel. This cookware is lightweight and cooks evenly.

Anodized aluminum. It's versatile, relatively easy to clean, and doesn't react to acidic foods like plain aluminum pots and pans do.

Copper-coated. A favorite of chefs, these pans help food to cook evenly; if you have copper with a stainless steel interior, even better.

Cast iron. The iron is so thick it generates the most, and most evenly distributed, heat. A little bit of iron, an important nutrient, leaches into food . . . which is a *good* thing. (Just avoid cooking really acidic foods like tomatoes, unless the pan is well seasoned, since iron doesn't react well with them.) To prevent rusting, the skillet should be seasoned frequently with oil—then heated until smoke starts to appear—and shouldn't be washed with strong detergents.

Enamel-coated iron. Safe to cook with according to the FDA's Center for Food Safety and Applied Nutrition, this variety is another foodie favorite.

As for baking, the same rules apply: No to Teflon, yes to stainless steel, aluminum, copper, and cast iron. Also, silicone baking molds are safe to use: Silicone is an inert material that won't transfer to foods during cooking.

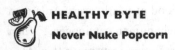

HEALTHY BYTE

Never Nuke Popcorn

Those bewitching buttery kernels have an ugly side: The lining of microwave popcorn bags are a source of PFOA, the same probable carcinogen found in Teflon. In tests, the FDA found that significant amounts of chemicals leach from the bags to the oil in the popcorn. Though the amounts from any single serving are small, PFOA remains in the body for years and levels can build up. On movie night, do your popping on the stove.

Step #10. Know Your Plastics

Despite the towering stacks of plastic containers most of us have accumulated, storing food in them is unadvisable, for many reasons. Plastics are made of petroleum, a nonrenewable resource, and during manufacturing chemicals such as benzene and dioxin are released into the air. Once you're done with it, a plastic container tossed into a landfill can take nearly a millennium to break down. But the major concern for our daily health is that some of the chemicals used to make plastic may leach into our food and drink.

There are different nasty chemicals to contend with. Two of the biggies: PVC, found in #3 containers, which leaches phthalates, a hormone disruptor; and Bisphenol A, a hormone-mimicking element found in #7 plastics (including water and baby bottles). Making safer choices about plastic food and liquid packaging is doable, if you know your numbers. The chasing-arrows recycling symbol, along with a number or letters, can be found on the bottom of most bottles and other containers. Cut back on plastics and choose your types wisely, and you'll reduce risks both personal and global.

✂ Copy and Carry ✂
Plastic by the Numbers

Here's a trick to remember which plastics are good and which are bad: Hold your hands in front of you. On your right hand (think: Right is right), all fingers but the middle (1, 2, 4, 5) are the safer plastics. What's on the left hand (6, 7) is bad.

PLASTICS TO AVOID

#3 PVC or V (polyvinyl chloride). The worst plastic for you and the environment. Commonly used in some cling wraps and food and liquid containers, this petroleum-based plastic can leach harmful chemicals, including phthalates, especially when in contact with oily or fatty foods, or during heating.

#6 PS (polystyrene). Used in Styrofoam containers; meat, egg, and bakery trays; and in its rigid form, clear take-out containers, plus some plastic cutlery and cups. Polystyrene may leach styrene into hot or acidic food it comes into contact with. Styrofoam also does not degrade in the environment, so it constitutes a big part of landfills.

#7 Other (usually polycarbonate). Used in five-gallon water bottles, clear plastic baby bottles, and metal can linings. Polycarbonate can release its primary building block, the hormonally disruptive Bisphenol A, into the liquid it contains.

SAFER PLASTICS

#1 PETE or PET (polyethylene terephthalate). Used for most clear beverage bottles and ketchup and salad dressing bottles.

#2 HDPE (high-density polyethylene). Most commonly found in "cloudy" jugs for milk, water, and juice; yogurt and spreadable butter tubs plus trash and grocery bags.

#4 LDPE (low-density polyethylene). Found in some squeezable bottles and frozen food storage bags.

#5 PP (polypropylene). Used in rigid containers, including some baby bottles and cups and bowls.

Store food in glass. The leftovers that sit in that plastic Chinese take-out container may be quietly sopping up chemicals from it. Glassware is durable and safe; stainless steel, ceramic, and porcelain also work well for food storage. (For recommended brands, see Healthy Resources.)

Never heat food in plastic. It causes chemicals to migrate into your meal. Nor should you microwave milk or formula in baby bottles. Remove plastic wrap from a plate or bowl before nuking. Use glass or ceramic dishes for serving warm food or beverages.

Limit canned food. Many aluminum cans, including those for liquid baby formula, are lined with polycarbonate plastic, which contains BPA. Opt for fresh and frozen foods, or powdered versions of baby formula.

Don't get stuck on cling wrap. Wax paper and butcher paper are safer alternatives to cling wrap, which is often made with PVC. (If you do use cling wrap, don't let it touch the food.) However, some wraps are now being made with low-density polyethylene (LDPE), which, though a bit less clingy, is not known to contain traces of potentially harmful additives.

Find a better bottle. Americans throw out more than 30 million plastic bottles per day; most of these are the ubiquitous PET #1 bottles which, while posing no immediate health risk, degrade and leach harmful chemicals when heated—a reason not to leave them in a hot, sunny car or buy them from vendors' bins exposed to the sun. And don't reuse these water bottles, as the plastic can erode upon repeated fillings. Reusable polycarbonate (#7) bottles aren't ideal either, since they contain BPA. In 2007, Mountain Equipment Co-op, Canada's largest specialty outdoor-goods retailer, pulled from its shelves most food and beverage containers made of polycarbonate plastic, like the ubiquitous Nalgene bottles, citing concern over possible health risks. If you love yours, just make sure you wash it by hand with a mild dishwashing soap, not in the dishwasher where the plastic can wear down.

A healthier option—cool-looking, too—is a reusable, virtually indestructible, aluminum or stainless steel bottle, like SIGG or Klean Kanteen. See Healthy Resources for more brands.

And a better baby bottle. In 2007, the advocacy group Environment California released their "Toxic Baby Bottles" report demonstrating how, when heated, five of the most popular brands made of polycarbonate—the clear, shatterproof plastic—leached BPA at levels found to harm lab animals. Safer baby bottles are made of cloudy plastic such as polyethylene (#1), polyethersulfone (PES), polyamide (PA), or polypropylene (#5). Or you could try tempered glass baby bottles that don't break as easily as regular glass. For recommended baby bottle brands, see Healthy Resources. Also, opt for clear silicone nipples (and pacifiers), which are made of a more stable and safer material than the yellow rubber or latex ones.

Expert Opinion
"Polluted" Breast Milk: Is Bottle-feeding Better?
By Sandra Steingraber, Ph.D., author of Having Faith: An Ecologist's Journey to Motherhood

One of the most important decisions you'll make as a new parent is how you will feed your baby. Stories in the media about the chemical contamination of human milk have made many mothers wonder if bottle-feeding might be an equally healthy alternative to breast-feeding. It is not.

The choice is clear: Our own breast milk is, hands down, the best food for your baby—far better than infant formula. This is the conclusion I reached after more than two years of studying data on the chemical contamination of breast milk.

Breast milk is not just food. It is also medicine. It swarms with antibodies and white blood cells drawn from your own body. By drinking it, your infant comes to share your immune system, and benefits mightily from it. Breast-fed infants have lower rates of hospitalization and death; develop fewer respiratory infections, gastrointestinal infections, urinary tract infections, ear infections, and meningitis; succumb less often to sudden infant death syndrome; and produce more antibodies in response to immunizations. Studies also consistently show that children who were breast-fed as infants suffer less from allergies, asthma, diabetes, colitis, and rheumatoid arthritis; have higher IQ scores; and are less likely to develop obesity and cancer.

Breast-feeding also protects mom's health. You will bleed less after childbirth; lose less blood during the chaotic days of early motherhood, because breast-feeding suppresses menstruation; be at lower risk for hip fracture after menopause; and have lower rates of ovarian and breast cancer.

There are logistical benefits, too. Breast-feeding can be done one-handed. Breast milk is so digestible that comparatively little comes out the other end. Less poop. And it has a less offensive odor. Really.

Then again, the chemical contamination of breast milk is not a trivial issue. When it comes to persistent organic pollutants, breast milk is the most contaminated of all human foods. It typically carries concentrations of organochlorine pollutants, such as dioxin, PCBs, and DDT, that are ten to twenty times higher than those in cow's milk. Other common contaminants of mother's milk include flame retardants, pesticides, wood preservatives, toilet deodorizers, and dry-cleaning fluids. And children who were breast-fed as babies have higher levels of chemical contaminants in their bodies than those who were formula-fed. (In spite of this fact, breast-fed children tend to be healthier and less prone to cancer.)

To provide your baby with the best nutrition possible:

1. Breast-feed. Your milk is unsubstitutable. Your baby needs it and will thrive on it.

2. Continue to avoid home and garden pesticides after your pregnancy. These chemicals can easily find their way into your milk through breathing and skin contact.

3. Eat healthy by choosing a low-contaminant diet. Eat organic and steer clear of fish high in mercury and PCBs.

4. Continue to avoid dry-cleaning fumes and solvents from paints, finishes, glues, and other building products.

5. Support efforts to phase out any and all toxic chemicals that accumulate in mother's milk. To help, contact Making Our Milk Safe (MOMS) at safemilk.org.

 ONE STEP BEYOND

Join a CSA. If you're willing to part with approximately three hundred to six hundred dollars up front (for a family of four), you'll get twenty weeks' worth of gorgeous, farm-fresh, in-season, often organic fruits and vegetables, bagged and ready to go, each week for most of the summer and fall. Sound delicious? Does it taste even better knowing you're helping to support a local farmer? The movement, more than one thousand farms strong nationwide, is called Community Supported Agriculture (CSA), and provides you with superior produce for what you pay at the supermarket or less—though if you simply can't consume that much per week, find a friend and halve your cost. Sites to help you find the farmers' market or CSA nearest you: ams.usda.gov/farmersmarkets; localharvest.org; foodroutes.org.

Grow your own. All it takes is a container, sun, and TLC to grow organic tomatoes, beans, or herbs. For more information on how to grow what you eat—even on a window ledge in the city—see Chapter 6.

CHAPTER 4

The Beauty Part

NATURAL BODY CARE

I s there anything more scrumptious than your kids freshly bathed—the day's playground grime and dinner crumbs washed down the drain, their hair combed, soft fingertips wrinkled by the bath water? And yet, if conventional soaps and creams are being used on them, they may not be making a clean getaway.

Most body products and toiletries are filled with unhealthy ingredients. Thanks to a major loophole in federal law, the $50 billion-a-year cosmetics industry routinely pumps synthetic chemicals into personal care items—for preservatives, color, fragrance, and suds making—without testing or monitoring them for long-term health effects on adults, let alone children, whose developing bodies are even more vulnerable to chemical harm. Manufacturers reason that it's okay to put these chemicals into personal care products, because each bottle contains only the tiniest amount. But think about how many products you use each day: shampoo, hair gel, body wash, deodorant, facial moisturizer, lotion, fragrance, skin prescriptions, mouthwash, makeup. According to the Environmental Working Group (EWG), the average person's grooming routine brings them into contact with 126 different chemicals each day. Also, the skin is very porous, absorbing up to 60 percent of what's put on it—and many of these chemicals enter the bloodstream directly. Put in those terms, it should be clear how the impact can add up over a year, certainly over a lifetime. Precautionary principle, anyone?

If, after reading this chapter, you feel the urge to purge every product on your shelf—as I did the moment we found out Jessica was pregnant—take a step back. It doesn't make practical, or environmental, sense to throw *all* those bottles and vials into the trash. It's okay to keep some of your favorites as you look for healthier substitutes. Also, a few products are simply irreplaceable, and that's fine, too (try getting a woman to part with her most trusted face cream—I've been there!). The idea is to start making better choices, not to drive yourself into a chemical-free frenzy. Here are some steps to help you evaluate the ingredients in your every-day grooming routine, and their safety to your family. For a list of recommended brands, see Healthy Resources.

Parentblog
Pay Now or Pay Later
By Vanessa Williams, actress

I've been a vegetarian and a devotee of holistic medicine for years. But nothing prepared me for the article I read online one night about all the harmful toxic chemicals that are in our cosmetics and shampoos. I was like, "Oh my god, we're getting cancer through the shampoo!" I stood up, walked to the bathroom, and just started tossing bottles and jars. I was trying to get rid of everything in my house that had sodium lauryl sulfates, parabens, and other chemicals which, until five minutes before, I'd never heard of or thought about. I felt I had no alternative. I could not unlearn what I'd just read.

Now, I love suds as much as the next person. I grew up on "Make it squeaky clean!" So this was no easy feat. Some of those products I'd used for years. And I cringed to think of having to now throw out a twelve-dollar bottle of shampoo. I couldn't bring myself to give them away to other people, either; I didn't want to be like, "Here, *you* take my toxins!"

Throwing out everything may sound dramatic, but for me, making a clean sweep was the only way to go. No matter how conscientious we may be about what goes in and on our bodies, we're exposed to so many harmful substances every day I just couldn't knowingly take that chance with my health and that of my family. One resource that helped me was the Environmental Working Group's "Skin Deep" report, which you can find online and which lists all the chemicals in your personal care products. The process was traumatizing. I went through my cosmetics; out went everything that came up on their hazardous list. When you're wearing heavy makeup daily and in front of the camera, you're especially vulnerable. Finding replacements hasn't been as challenging as I'd feared, though. I believe that sooner rather than later supply will meet demand for the healthier choices we continue to make.

But too many Americans seem to miss the connection between all this toxic exposure and illness, an awareness that what we put in and on our bodies directly affects our health. People tend to be slaves to their taste buds and to convenience, and don't get that their habits exacerbate their exposure to cancer, stroke, and all manner of diseases.

I am acutely concerned about this because in my community, the African-American community, we're more likely to get diseases in disproportionate numbers, and more likely to die from them—diseases like type 2 diabetes that are 100 percent preventable and reversible by changes in diet, exercise, and attitude. Recent studies conclude that breast cancer is growing most rapidly among African-American women. Many close friends and family members have been affected by these illnesses. Losing their breasts, their uteruses, their colons, their lives—it's not for no reason. After my epiphany, I was on the path to do whatever I could to make my life even greener and healthier. I started using exclusively nontoxic cleaners in my kitchen, bathroom, and laundry. Living as we do, perhaps there's no way to avoid toxic chemicals altogether. But taking action to reduce our risk is imperative; that's where nutrition comes in.

My family and I have made the decision to live long, healthy lives, and every choice we make informs that. Granted, some of these choices can be more costly in the short term; health-food store prices are often higher than at traditional supermarkets. I know that when money is tight, two dollars makes a significant difference. But I ask myself, Is it worth it to pay a couple of dollars more for this dishwashing liquid and avoid the risk of poisoning myself and my family? Absolutely! When folks complain, I tell them that either you pay now or you pay later: in doctors' bills, or the inconvenience and trauma of having to have your breasts removed, or your foot amputated because your diabetes is at a point where there's no alternative.

You have to be the expert in your own life on the health of your family. It's a lifelong learning process. It's not too much to ask. You're worth it.

Step #1. Read the Fine Print

Labels on beauty and body care products are hard to decode for even the most diligent consumer. Companies are free to slap on an ORGANIC, NATURAL, or HYPOALLERGENIC label without claims to back them up, thanks to loopholes in the government's oversight of the personal care industry. Just because a soap or shampoo contains some natural or plant-derived ingredients doesn't mean it's free of chemicals or synthetics. And "natural" doesn't necessarily mean safer: Some herbal ingredients cause allergic reactions, rashes, and worse.

I know this all sounds confusing. Perhaps more than any other topic in this book, the safety of personal care products creates bewilderment and frustration. To become a savvy consumer, you're going to have to learn a few terms and study ingredient lists. Bring your glasses; play detective! With a little diligence, you'll find products you're happy with. And when you do, tell a few friends—they'll be grateful that you could help them with their own sleuthing.

One place to start: the U.S. Department of Agriculture's green-and-white CERTIFIED ORGANIC label, the same one you see on cereal boxes. It has now been extended to cover personal care products, too. This is the rare label you can trust; it means that at least 70 percent of ingredients found in the product must be organic. Even better: the USDA seal that says 100 PERCENT ORGANIC.

Another clue is to check whether the manufacturer has signed a compact started by the Campaign for Safe Cosmetics, a coalition of public and environmental health groups that lobbies companies to voluntarily eliminate chemicals linked to cancer, birth defects, and other health problems, and to promote the use of certified organic and natural ingredients. For a list of companies that have signed on, see safecosmetics.org.

The bottom line? Keep it simple. Start with the things you use a lot and look for a straightforward ingredients list. The more pronounceable the words, the better. If the label is a string of scientific gibberish, ask yourself if you or your child needs the product at all.

100
percentage of women of child-bearing age with phthalates in their bodies, likely due to cosmetic use. (Centers for Disease Control and Prevention, 2005)

0
number of epidemiological studies examining impact of phthalates on human fetal development (prompting the American Academy of Pediatrics to call for activism and research on the chemicals).

 HEALTHY BYTE
How Does Your Face Cream Rate?

Curious to know how good-for-you your favorite body products are? Considering a new one? Log on to the "Skin Deep" report, a searchable database of ingredients found in nearly twenty-five thousand products, created by the Environmental Working Group at cosmeticsdatabase.com. See how each rates on a 1–10 scale from Healthy to Hazardous, and which health issues the ingredients are linked to.

Step # 2. Lose the Scent

We get attached to the smell of our body products: that green-apple shampoo, a spicy perfume, the marshmallow scent of baby skin cream. But most of these intoxicating aromas are phony—chemical concoctions that can trigger allergic reactions and respiratory ailments, including asthma. And many fragrances contain hidden ingredients that might pose chronic long-term health risks.

For instance, most conventional perfumes, hair gels, shampoos, and other scented products contain the family of fragrance-carrying chemicals called phthalates, which have been proven to interfere with hormonal and reproductive function in animals—and, in one small study, were linked to reproductive abnormalities in baby boys exposed to high levels in utero. (Keep in mind that research on this topic is only preliminary and the health repercussions are not well understood.) In a 2002 report by the EWG, phthalates were found in nearly three-quarters of the seventy-two personal care products it tested. The number of brands that listed the ingredient on their label? Zero. That's because the hundreds of chemicals that go into making a fragrance are considered "trade secrets" and don't have to be identified on the packaging; the label can simply say "fragrance."

1,100+
number of chemical ingredients banned from cosmetics in the European Union.

9
number of banned ingredients in the United States (Not Just a Pretty Face: The Ugly Side of the Beauty Industry by Stacy Malkan)

Another reason to avoid artificial fragrances: Most fake scents are made from petrochemicals and give off vapors (VOCs) like those that waft from products such as paint strippers and cleaning products. For that reason, they carry the same health risks (cancer, liver damage), too.

Switch to fragrance-free products with naturally based ingredients and fewer synthetic additives, especially in children's products where the tempting berry and bubblegum scents might fool some kids into thinking they're edible. Read the ingredients list closely, since some products labeled UNSCENTED may in fact contain other chemicals to mask the chemical smells. Another bewildering paradox, I know. But the bottom line: If it says FRAGRANCE, put it down. Many safer products are also naturally scented with organic essential oils (extracted from a plant's flowers, leaves, and stems) such as almond and lavender. Some people are allergic to essential oils, so first do a patch test on skin before use.

Step #3. Find Better Bubbles

We tend to equate supersudsiness with cleanliness. However, bubbles that froth out of conventional soaps and shampoos expose your family to some strong chemical detergents that help remove dirt and oil. By far the most common of these are sodium laureth sulfate (SLES) and its chemical cousin, sodium lauryl sulfate (SLS); they're the foaming agents in nearly every sudsy product in the house—shampoos, bath bubbles, bar soaps, as well as laundry and dishwasher detergents. They also make skin more permeable. While SLS and SLES are considered safe by the FDA, the worry is that they can interact with other product ingredients to form carcinogens. Fortunately SLS-free products now abound on the market.

One more thing to keep in mind: Children's shampoos and bubble baths will often tout how "gentle" and "hypoallergenic" they are, but those claims tell you nothing about what's inside the bottle; they just mean the manufacturer thinks their formula's gentler than others. Most regular kids' shampoos contain as many harsh additives as do adults', including detanglers, thickeners, and synthetic colors and fragrances. Just another reason why organic and natural brands are the way to go. Consult the EWG's Parent's Safety Guide to Children's Personal Care Products found at cosmeticsdatabase.com/special/parentsguide.

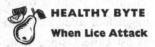

HEALTHY BYTE
When Lice Attack

Each year, roughly 6 million elementary school kids are beset with pediculosis, or head lice. The conventional way to treat head lice is with prescription shampoos such as Kwell, which contains a powerful, nerve-attacking insecticide that has even been reported to cause seizures in some children, and Nix, which contains a mildly toxic insecticide.

Nits themselves—unhatched eggs attached to the hair shaft—spread like crazy once they hatch, so act before it gets out of hand. The most crucial part of a lice-removal program is a thorough combing. The University of Pittsburgh Cancer Institute Center for Environmental Oncology (environmentaloncology.org) recommends the following treatment:

If you see nits or lice on your child's head, wash hair with either a coconut oil Castile soap mixed with a few drops of naturally insecticidal tea tree and neem oil (available in health-food stores—but note that many such oils are toxic if ingested) or a shampoo made with tea tree oil (ten drops of tea tree oil to one ounce shampoo). Rinse and rewash with the same mixture, but don't rinse again—yet. Instead, wrap a towel around the soapy head and wait half an hour, *then* rinse. Comb clean hair with a normal comb, then comb again thoroughly with a metal, nit-removing comb (with close-set teeth). Proceed chunk by chunk until all nits are gone. Rewash and rinse the hair; check one last time for nits. Repeat the process every few days for at least two weeks.

You'll also want to clean your child's towels, bedding, and clothes in hot water and dry them on high heat for an hour. Place toys and stuffed animals in plastic bags and keep sealed for two weeks to kill lice. Replace all hair utensils; vacuum carpets.

You can also try this shower cap trick (from the Washington State Department of Health): Saturate hair with olive oil or full-fat mayonnaise, don a shower cap, and leave it on for two to four hours. Shampoo the oils out and use a vinegar rinse (½ cup vinegar + ½ cup water) to loosen nits so they're easier to comb out.

For more natural lice remedies and information, see environmentaloncology.org, headlice.org, and liceout.com.

Get the dope on your soap. Bar soaps are typically made from sodium tallowate, a combination of lye and cow or sheep fat, and then goosed up with more of the same detergents, fragrance, preservatives, and alcohol dyes found in shampoo.

It's easy—very easy—to get around using chemically infused soaps. Look for natural, handmade, and even locally produced soaps, widely available in health-food stores, pharmacies, and at farmers' markets. Castile soap is just a term for soap made from plant oil (such as olive, coconut, hemp, and almond); these come in liquids and bars and are another healthy choice, as are natural glycerin soaps (not to be confused with synthetic glycerin bars, which contain some of the same chemicals as regular soaps).

Note to germophobes: Antibacterial soaps are *totally unnecessary*. In fact, they're a terrible idea: They're filled with harmful antimicrobial pesticides such as triclosan. Research shows that washing your hands with regular soap and water work perfectly well for loosening dirt and germs. The important thing is the friction from rubbing your hands together, and doing it long enough—get your kids to sing the alphabet while washing.

Finally, if you're bathing your kids every single day, regardless of how dirty they get, you may want to reconsider. According to the hygiene hypothesis, the recent leaps in asthma and eczema rates can be partly explained by our cultural insistence on hypercleanliness and germ eradication. (One recent study by England's Bristol University investigated how frequently eleven thousand toddlers were bathed, showered, or had their hands washed every day, and found that "increased levels of hygiene" were linked to higher rates of asthma and eczema for kids aged between two and four.) The theory holds that children raised in less sterile environments are exposed to more bacteria and infections that prime their immune systems and protect them from disease. Of course, kids who get very dirty playing outdoors are reaping the benefits of exposure anyway; a parent can certainly be excused for having them wash the grime off before bedtime.

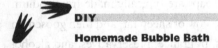

DIY

Homemade Bubble Bath

Commercial bubble bath is often the cause of bubble bath cystitis, a painful irritation of a child's urethra. Here's a chance to prevent problems by using a more natural solution.

½ cup glycerin
1 quart water

1 bar (4 ounces) Castile soap or liquid form
5–10 drops of essential oil for fragrance

Mix glycerin and water. Dissolve soap (heating the water/glycerin mixture or shaving the soap will help dissolve it). Add essential oil. Shake well when mixing and again just before use. Note: Castile soap is very mild and made from olive oil. Glycerin is a natural, nonoily moisturizer. All ingredients are readily available at department stores, supermarkets, pharmacies, and online.

—*from* What's Toxic, What's Not *by Dr. Gary Ginsberg and Brian Toal, M.S.P.H.*

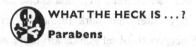

WHAT THE HECK IS . . . ?
Parabens

Parabens are a family of preservatives that turn up a lot in personal care products. Lately they've generated lots of controversy. In one study from Brunel University in England, researchers linked parabens to the possibility that male babies exposed in utero could have lower sperm counts. Another recent British study found traces of parabens in the breast cancer cells of women. Many cosmetics manufacturers use parabens—variations include methylparaben, propylparaben, or butylparaben—to kill bacteria, giving the product a prolonged shelf life. Although parabens' long-term health effects are far from proven, there is evidence to warrant caution. As with any chemical additives, it's best to avoid them if possible, especially in babies' and children's shampoos, wipes, and sunscreens. Pregnant women should also skip them. For paraben-free skin-care lines, see Healthy Resources.

Step # 4. Oil Your Engine, Not Your Skin

Petroleum and mineral oil, both derived from fossil fuels, are common basic ingredients in cosmetics, particularly lotions, foundations, cleansers, lipsticks, and lip balms. Propylene glycol, a chemical additive that carries moisture in cosmetics, comes from petroleum, while petroleum distillates, possible human carcinogens, are found in several U.S. brands of mascara and other products. (Look for the terms *petroleum* or *liquid paraffin*.) Most of the fragrances in these products also come from crude oil, as do parabens. The long-term health effects of petroleum products are not yet known, but we have some hint of their potency from other applications. (Propylene glycol is also an ingredient in antifreeze and paint!)

Even beauty experts who aren't particularly green often encourage people with sensitive skin to use water-based rather than petroleum-based lotions and creams, because oil can lock moisture against the skin, blocking pores. That's all the more reason to seek water-based formulas made with naturally derived moisturizers like shea butter and jojoba. Same goes for kids and teens, especially as they enter that dark tunnel of self-awareness known as adolescence. Since youthful oil glands are more active than adults,' teens may not need to moisturize anyway, but you can help them pick out a non-petroleum-based cream if they need it during drier winter months.

Baby skin (apart from the business end) arguably doesn't need moisturizing, either. Even mild baby creams can dry out skin and contain fragrance that may be sensitizing. In the dry dregs of winter, though, after a bath choose natural oils like olive, almond, apricot kernel, and avocado. Or use vegetable glycerin, shea butter, or soy lecithin.

🍐 HEALTHY BYTE: FEED YOUR FACE
By Carolyn Murphy, model, actress, activist

I grew up in Florida and learned from my mother to use many of the fruits and vegetables that grew all around us for healthy skin care. We used to squish avocado and olive oil onto our faces if they were dehydrated, or make an oatmeal and honey face mask. We'd mash bougainvillea blossoms to make shampoo and rinse our hair with vinegar to strip residue from conventional shampoos. This wasn't always practical, but it was really fun. And judging from the fact that my skin ended up being a major asset in my career, it clearly worked. Here are two of my mom's favorite recipes. Mix, slather, enjoy:

To exfoliate. If you're dry and flaky, combine 2 egg whites, a tablespoon of milk, and a tablespoon of honey. Leave on face for a few minutes; rinse.

To hydrate. Mix avocado and a little bit of milk and oatmeal made from rolled oats. Leave on for a few minutes; rinse.

Step # 5. Dispel Diaper Rash Safely

Diaper creams too often contain petroleum products (as in petroleum jelly or Vaseline), fragrances, parabens, and other unwanted chemicals. To prevent diaper rash, keep vulnerable areas dry and expose to fresh air as much as possible. If redness develops, zinc diaper cream made without harsh chemicals usually takes care of it. Other good rash home remedies: cornstarch and aloe vera gel (don't use them both at once, though—you're liable to make muffins!).

Nix the talc. Never use talcum baby powder for bottom blotting—or any other purpose. Your mom may have rolled you in it like she was flouring dough, but talc can irritate the lungs when inhaled and there is evidence that talc may be contaminated with traces of illness-causing asbestos.

Skip the chemical baby wipes. Conventional wipes are often soaked with alcohol, fragrances, and other skin irritants. For the first few weeks of a baby's life, use a water-saturated paper towel or cloth, eventually moving on to wipes that are unbleached and free of dyes and fragrances. Keep a pump thermos filled with warm water mixed with a teaspoon of baking soda on hand to save time and water while cleaning.

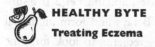 **HEALTHY BYTE**
Treating Eczema

The most common cause of eczema rashes in babies is food allergies, from their diet or that of their nursing mother. This itchy skin inflammation may also be triggered by irritation from harsh soaps, detergents, or synthetic finishes on clothing. Eruptions are commonly treated with frequent lubrication of the skin, reduced soap exposure, diet changes, and occasionally with a short course of a steroid cream, such as hydrocortisone.

Prevention is key. Work with your pediatrician to evaluate what, if any, food allergen might be in your baby's diet. Avoid wool, overheating, and slathering your child with creams containing fragrances or other harsh additives. Use mild laundry detergent. And keep skin moist with a daily rubdown of a light oil (like almond, sesame, or olive).

Step #6. Be Sunscreen Smart

Reality check: Skin cancer is the most common cancer in the United States: An estimated 40 to 50 percent of Americans who live to age sixty-five will get it at least once. Covering up with hats, shirts, and beach umbrellas is the best way to protect your skin and that of your kids from the sun's potent ultraviolet rays. But unless you're prepared to sport burkhas to the pool, you're going to need sunscreen, so be sure it's a good one.

The Environmental Working Group (EWG) recently published an investigation into 831 name-brand sunscreens and discovered that many are neither safe nor effective. Consider this doozy: One in eight high-SPF sunscreens does not protect from UVA radiation, the rays linked to skin damage, aging, and potentially skin cancer. Furthermore, many sunscreens contain phthalates, parabens, and other estrogen-like compounds. Fortunately, the EWG identified 135 health-safe products that offer very good sun protection. (Go to cosmeticsdatabase.com and click on sunscreens.) Here's what you need to know:

Look for "full spectrum" protection. The safest and most effective sunscreens protect against both UVA *and* UVB rays and form an actual barrier between your skin and sunlight. Ingredients to look for: zinc oxide and titanium dioxide.

Go for a high SPF. The American Cancer Society recommends a sunscreen with an SPF of at least 15. Higher SPFs offer more protection, but above SPF 30, there's not much difference. Most important, coat the skin, or sunscreen isn't effective—and reapply frequently (especially on the face, shoulders, neck, forearms, hands, and feet) as the lotion breaks down in the sun and comes off in water, even when "waterproof." Test sunscreen on a patch of soft skin on the inside of your child's arm before applying, as kids' skin is especially sensitive to chemical allergens. And don't forget to slather on the stuff before sending them off to school, camp, or to play sports; most exposure comes through brief episodes.

Embrace the pale. Skip tanning salons—it's especially important to get the message through to tan-worshipping teens: The UV radiation of a tanning bed is up to fifteen times stronger than the sun's. And the chemicals in self-tanning products have not been tested adequately for safety.

Sun and bugs don't mix. Avoid combination sunscreen/insect repellents: Sunscreen is most effective when applied every two hours, but replenishing insect repellent so often could lead to overexposure.

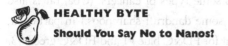 **HEALTHY BYTE**
Should You Say No to Nanos?

Nanoparticles have been quietly turning up in many body care products, especially sunscreen (nanos turn white creams like zinc oxide clear when spread on skin). Nanotechnology involves the manipulation of materials at the atomic scale, so the resulting bits are minuscule. The worry is that nanos are small enough not just to pass through skin but also to penetrate body tissue and organs, potentially causing harm. Several environmental groups are deeply concerned about the lack of labeling (the package won't alert you to their presence) or reliable safety information, and have called for more research. However, in its big-effort sunscreen evaluation, the EWG found that nano-containing zinc and titanium products were among the most protective on the market. So the jury is still out; if you prefer to avoid nanoparticles in your sunscreen, the EWG database (cosmeticsdatabase.com) lists products that contain them.

Step # 7. Forget To-Dye-For Hair

Women who frequently color their hair often wonder whether their dyes and treatments are safe. Some studies have found no risk at all. However, one recent University of Southern California study found that women using permanent hair dye at least once a month for a year or longer more than double their risk of bladder cancer. Another study, from the Yale University School of Medicine, found that long-term use of permanent hair dyes may increase risk for non-Hodgkins lymphoma. These are good arguments to exert caution.

The chemicals found in many hair dyes and perms run to the heavy-duty end of the spectrum. Oxidation dyes—used to lighten hair—usually contain hydrogen peroxide (which is safe) and ammonia (which is not). Dyes that darken hair, called progressive dyes, may rely on lead acetate to do the job, which contains—yes—lead. Permanent coal-tar dyes found in seventy-one common hair dye products tested by the EWG have been linked to some types of cancers. (Coal tar is also found in some dandruff shampoos.) In particular, watch out for FD&C blue #1 and FD&C green #3.

11
percentage of the 10,000+ chemical ingredients found in cosmetics that have been assessed for health and safety by the Cosmetic Ingredient Review, an industry-funded panel of scientists. (Environmental Working Group, 2004)

As for perms and straighteners, the solutions used to curl hair contain chemicals that are irritating to skin and lungs, and harmful if they get in the eyes; meanwhile, hair straighteners can burn skin and some even contain Teflon-like additives.

The bottom line: Less is more! The less hair dye and perm chemicals used over a lifetime, the less likely a person will be exposed to levels high enough to raise a health risk.

Most important, doctors exhort pregnant and nursing women to skip perms and single-process hair dyes to avoid passing chemicals along to the baby. Highlights are no doubt safer, since the dye coats the hair shaft and doesn't touch the skin. So if your teen comes home with a pink streak in her ponytail, it's no cause for alarm (from a health standpoint, that is!).

There are plenty of color treatments that use gentler, natural ingredients, such as those made from henna, which is herb-derived and runs the ruddy spectrum from brown to orange. Eco-beauty lines also produce natural color products (see Healthy Resources).

Parentblog
You're in Charge
By Kate Hudson, actress, entrepreneur

When it comes to living a healthier life, I really feel you have to call your own shots. You have to begin by deciding to make positive changes. I started by making certain things myself. I've made lotions, candles, homeopathic remedies, and aromatherapy treatments, mainly as fun hobbies that then developed my interest in the types of ingredients used in products and their effects on us and the environment. This kick started me to develop a business. I found it wasn't so easy to find truly natural hair care products so my hairdresser and I started a line of them—David Babaii for WildAid. They're free of parabens, sulfates, and animal products. There's no animal testing, plus a portion of the money goes to protecting endangered species and their habitats. We're planning to expand into other body and home products, which will include body, face, baby products, etc.

Food is another area that is important to me. Cooking is one of my favorite things to do; when I'm away on a set and can't cook for Ryder, it drives me crazy. I like to get as inventive as possible. Jessica Seinfeld beat me to the punch with her book because I hide good things in Ryder's food all the time. He doesn't like veggies so I boil them, puree them, then hide them in anything so he doesn't say, *Mommy, I see something green...* Often

I put it in lasagna or other kinds of pasta. I'll put flaxseed oil or a flavored omega-3 in natural peanut butter.

It's all about taking charge. You can't stop your child from what he's going to do outside the home. But I can do something—quite a lot, actually—about the products *in* my home. That requires my being as conscious about things as possible. Plus, I believe in constantly finding new ways to do things—myself.

Step #8. Put a Nail in Your Polish Habit

Simply put: Reduce your use of standard nail polish. It contains several harmful chemicals, including formaldehyde (partly responsible for the eye-watering fumes), acetone, and phthalates, which make polish chip-resistant. Phthalates, which mimic estrogen, are banned from cosmetics in Europe; fortunately, some American manufacturers—including a few of the biggies like L'Oréal and Revlon—have begun removing them from their polishes. Pregnant women should definitely opt for a phthalate-free polish; teens and girls, too. Next time you get a manicure, BYOB (bottle, that is). If you do your polish at home, make sure it's in a well-ventilated space.

Or try this polishless manicure: File nails, soak fingers, then shape cuticles with a nut oil or olive oil. Dry hands and buff nails with a chamois cloth.

Parentblog
Message in a Bottle
By Josie Maran, model, founder of Josie Maran Cosmetics

I started modeling when I was twelve. It was fun dressing up; I liked the fantasy of playing so many different characters. I also really appreciated the artistry of the makeup and wearing it gave me confidence. But I broke out a lot, which taught me that it wasn't good to pile on so many products every single day. At some point, a friend had given me a little bottle of Argan oil, which comes from the nut of an ancient Moroccan tree. I fell in love with it; now it's the only thing I use on my face and skin. I wanted to get the word out, and I wanted to find out what other cosmetics could be made without synthetic chemicals. I took some of my favorites to a lab and asked if they could make natural versions. That's how my company was born.

Since I had my daughter, Rumi, I use 100 percent organic products as much as I can. Sometimes that means going without deodorant, but I've tried to make it cool to stink. I've embraced it and I've gotten my friends to do it as well.

Throughout my career, my family said, *Come on, Josie, do something.* I always knew I wanted to affect change—my grandmother teaches human rights activism at UC Berkeley, and my dad's a green builder, after all—but I didn't have any direction. Finally, something just clicked, and it was easy to act.

Step #9. Make Over Your Makeup

Cosmetics are starting to get their own natural overhaul. Products that carry a 100 PERCENT ORGANIC or 75 PERCENT ORGANIC label are lower in (or devoid of) unhealthy chemicals such as synthetic dyes, artificial fragrances, and petrochemicals. Organic or all-natural makeup—including face powder; foundation; and lip, cheek, and eye color—are derived from naturally occurring mineral pigments and organic plant extracts, plus oils and waxes, so they're gentle and less reactive with sensitive skin than the conventional stuff. There are several lines now available that conform to these high standards. See the EWG's "Skin Deep" database (and Healthy Resources) for brands.

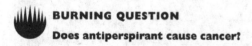 **BURNING QUESTION**
Does antiperspirant cause cancer?

A few years ago, a widely circulated e-mail stirred panic with the suggestion that the aluminum salts in antiperspirants could lead to breast cancer. (Piling on, another urban legend linked aluminum to Alzheimer's.) In a 2004 report, the National Cancer Institute disputed the claims, and to this day there is no scientific evidence supporting them. One thing that's *un*disputed: Most antiperspirants contain those pesky hormone-disrupting parabens, in the form of preservatives. Consider whether a product you use every day, in such an intimate place, should contain such an unwelcome active ingredient. Those who want to break a cleaner sweat can buy natural deodorant brands (the EWG has ranked some of these on cosmeticsdatabase.com). The Crystal (thecrystal.com) is made of natural mineral salts that work not by reducing perspiration but by making it difficult for bacteria—the main culprit in body odor—to survive in your armpit. Whatever product you use, aerosols should be avoided because of their use of propellants, which are linked to respiratory problems.

❧ Expert Opinion ❧
What They Don't Tell Us
*By Dr. Devra Davis, director, Center for Environmental Oncology,
University of Pittsburgh Cancer Institute; author of* The Secret History
of the War on Cancer

Here's a big myth we're battling: *Most cancer is inherited.*

Not true. But because of the misconception, people often think there's little we can do to protect ourselves. Only one in ten breast cancer cases occurs in a woman born with a genetic risk of the disease. Genetic predisposition accounts for no more than 20 percent of all childhood cancers. In fact, a large percentage of childhood cancers are due to environmental exposures, including those of their fathers and mothers *before* conception, and of their mothers during pregnancy. They are thus preventable. Cancer deaths are dropping chiefly because fewer people are smoking and we have improved the ability to find and treat cancers of the breast, cervix, and colon—in short, we're getting better at not dying of cancer because we're getting better at identifying and removing its causes.

Another myth: *A small amount of a chemical carcinogen in a children's product isn't dangerous because the level is so low.*

Not true. Life is a mixture. Cancer and other diseases can take decades to develop. Even if the levels of a single contaminant may be low, they add up over a lifetime. This is why known animal carcinogens like 1,4-dioxane are banned in European baby shampoos and bubble baths. American and Canadian childrens' bathing products do not ban these same materials.

Another myth: *The FDA protects us because they've established standards.*

Again, not true. David Steinman's research, discussed in his book *Safe Trip to Eden*, as well as other studies showed that at least 15 percent of cosmetic products contaminated with 1,4-dioxane exceed the FDA's recommended upper limit. But these "limits" are voluntary, and companies flouting them face no consequences from the federal government. Consumers have no way to know what the levels may be in products they purchase, because there is no monitoring, nor requirement for reporting on them.

What concerns me most is the insidious repackaging of information—the distorting, revising, concealing, and ignoring by corporations and the government. Thomas Jefferson said that democracy rests on an informed public that freely consents to be governed—but that assumes we're getting the proper information. And we're simply not. How can we consent when we don't even know they put toxic stuff in a product that we then rub on our babies' bottoms? People often ask me if I think the facts I report are just too alarming. I don't. We all have natural repair processes that keep us healthy much of the time. Getting informed about hazards we can avoid is critical to our health and that of our children and grandchildren. What I *do* find alarming is the volume of information that's been withheld from us, and how much we don't know because not enough study is being done on the controversial subjects. That's what people should be alarmed about, and what has to change.

Step #10. Flash a Healthy Smile

Starting in the 1950s, toothpaste manufacturers started adding fluoride to prevent tooth decay. And fluoride has proven very effective at that task, cutting down cavities by as much as half. Some health experts speculate that many of us already get more than enough of it through public drinking water (fluoride overload, or fluorosis, can in rare cases cause white spots on permanent teeth), but for now we don't know enough about the long-term health effects of fluoride to change our habits.

Still, because kids are more likely to swallow while brushing, there are reasons to buy natural toothpaste (many brands are also fluoride-fortified). For one, they don't contain the fake sweetener saccharin. They're also less likely to be pumped up with artifical flavors, preservatives, or colors. Many natural toothpastes rely on plant extracts, like peppermint and fennel, to freshen breath. If you live in a community where the water isn't fluoridated (if you drink well water, for instance), then your kids should definitely be using fluoridated toothpaste. If your tap water contains fluoride, it's probably okay to skip it during brushing.

 ONE STEP BEYOND

Sign up. Let companies know that their customers want safe products by signing the Safe Cosmetics petition at action.safecosmetics.org/petition.

Fill up. Buy reusable containers (especially glass!) and refill them with eco-friendly shampoos and lotions available in bulk in natural food stores.

Read up. Still want to know more? See *Unreasonable Risk: How to Avoid Cancer from Cosmetics and Personal Care* by Dr. Samuel Epstein. It will be one of your best allies in your search for healthier products.

CHAPTER 5

Child's Play

SAFER TOYS, GEAR, AND CLOTHING

P arenthood today has, to some degree, become about acquiring mounds of new stuff. A generation or two ago, kids would lie peacefully in cradles or play with a few handmade toys (or whatever items they could scrounge up around the house) while mom went about her business, with no beeping electrical pulses or lights to distract them. On one level much of this can be chalked up to advancement: Thank goodness for car seats with five-point harnesses; and, who knows, maybe those sound and light shows really do create baby Einsteins. But on another level this behavior is far from logical, since much of what we buy is made from hunks of plastic, which creates pollution in its manufacturing, may release fumes into the home, and sits in landfills until kingdom come.

The challenge for parents is to exert some restraint in what they buy for their kids—and for themselves. Many of the gadgets we feel we must have to simplify the tasks of parenting inevitably complicate things (wipes warmer, anyone?) and we too often end up acquiring toys and clothes that our kids don't need or even want that badly—or, even when they do, tire of quickly. These things clutter the house, collect dust and other allergens, contain chemicals our kids are at risk for ingesting (remember *l'affaire* Thomas the Tank Engine and the wave of toy recalls in

2007, mostly due to lead paint?) . . . and then they become landfill. I remember the panicky feeling of looking at a baby gift registry in the
weeks before Luke was born, wondering on one hand whether we'd
checked off enough stuff to be prepared for the frenzy of new parenthood, and on the other, feeling dismayed over the wastefulness, not to
mention anxious about how the heck we would find room for all our new
acquisitions. (We ended up scaling back our wish list and registering at a
green nursery purveyor—see the Healthy Resources section for names.
Also, a looming due date is a good excuse to throw a green-themed baby
shower, since you can exert greater control over what kind of gifts come
in. Flip to our blueprint for the Healthy Child version on page 32.)

I know I must sound like a killjoy. Yet the antidote is genuinely easy,
and a boon to the whole family. For one, buy less. For another, buy better: Introduce less stuff that might inadvertently compromise your children's developmental or physical health. Before you shop, ask yourself
why you're getting something. Is it wanted? Needed? Or has a marketer
convinced your child that he or she really wants and needs it? Either way,
here are some tips to help your kids play, dress, and ride safely.

Step #1. Seek Out PVC-free

The soft plastic used in so many cheap, colorful toys, especially PVC
(polyvinyl chloride) plastic, can release unhealthy fumes into the air
(known as "off-gassing"), exposing kids to inhalation. Soft plastic toys
are particularly troublesome—rubber ducks, bath books, plastic cars,
inflatable figures, dolls, and learning toys also contain phthalates, softening agents used to make PVC pliable, the same stuff used in vinyl
flooring. Studies have proven that phthalates can be hormonally disruptive in animals, and can easily leach out when kids suck or chew on a
toy, like flavor out of gum.

Another reason to be wary of PVC is that toys made of it may also
contain lead, which is sometimes used as a stabilizer in this kind of plastic. Kids can be exposed to lead when they put toys in their mouths, or
when they lick their hands while playing.

BURNING QUESTION
How do I clean scummy bath toys?

Bath toys are a breeding ground for bacteria and mold, especially those with holes in the bottom. You can squeeze water out of tub toys and hang them to dry in a netting bag; once a week, throw them in the dishwasher or submerge them for a few minutes in a solution of one part vinegar to three parts hot water. However, many squeeze toys are made with PVC, which you're best off avoiding. Kids can have fun in the tub with safer, less microbially prone objects—bowls, spoons, and airtight hard-plastic figures.

How do you avoid PVC? First, you need to identify it, which is easier said than done. On packaging, look for the #3 or the letters PVC next to the three-arrow recycling symbol. Look for "phthalate free" on the packaging; if a toy smells like a new shower curtain, it likely contains phthalates. You can always call the manufacturer's customer service line or check their Web site to investigate the materials they use. Fortunately more manufacturers are pledging to remove PVCs and phthalates and many already are phthalate free, including BRIO, IKEA, LEGO, Gerber, Little Tikes, Early Start, Sassy, and Tiny Love.

Binkys and teethers. Whether your baby takes a pacifier will be up to you, your pediatrician, and of course your infant, since not all babies show the same eagerness to suck. Nevertheless, most babies start shoving objects into their mouths around three or four months, both to soothe painful gums and as a way to explore the world. So the best thing we can do is to make sure that what they suck on won't bring harm.

Opt for clear silicone pacifiers over the yellow rubber ones, which may contain unwanted chemicals. And some teethers are made of PVC (#3): Despite the fact that the U.S. Consumer Product Safety Commission has asked American manufacturers to remove phthalates from baby pacifiers and teethers for children under three, many have not complied. Those that have include Chicco, Evenflo, Gerber, Sassy, Hasbro (Playskool), and Mattel (Fisher-Price), among others. One healthy teething idea: Dip the corner of a washcloth in apple juice and freeze it—the cold is soothing.

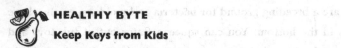

HEALTHY BYTE
Keep Keys from Kids

Keys make lousy pacifiers. Most brass keys contain lead in their alloys, and traces of lead can pass from hands to mouth. Make sure they wash hands after handling keys or digging in your purse for them.

Package deal. A 2007 national study of PVC packaging—that clear plastic casing enveloping toys and electronics, which requires either a Ph.D. or a machete to open—revealed that more than 60 percent of samples tested contained toxic heavy metals at levels that violate legal limits in nineteen states. Fortunately, many companies have committed to eliminating PVC packaging. For more information, see toxicsinpack aging.org.

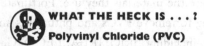

WHAT THE HECK IS . . . ?
Polyvinyl Chloride (PVC)

PVC is a material used in the manufacture of everything from pacifi-ers and water bottles to toys and shower curtains and vinyl flooring—typically in plastics with the #3 recycling designation. Made from the flammable gas vinyl chloride, a known human carcinogen, PVC re-leases vapors (a process called "off-gassing") that can be inhaled. PVC becomes a soft, squishy plastic when combined with softening agents called *phthalates*, which are often chewed on and ingested. Studies have linked some phthalates to hormone disruption in animals. Cut back on your kids' plastic toys to reduce their exposure. It's that sim-ple. At least fourteen countries and the European Union have banned phthalates in toys for children under three; meanwhile, the state of California has just adopted a ban, and other states and cities are ex-pected to follow.

Step #2. Get the Lead Out of the Toy Box

Recent toy recalls have made for unsettling headlines. The first nine months of 2007 saw a record fifty recalls due to lead exposure risk by the Consumer Product Safety Commission. Many of these were aimed at major manufacturers such as Fisher-Price, Mattel, and Disney, though all the contaminated products were made in China or elsewhere in Asia. In every case, the culprit was lead in the paint or coating. The concern? Lead can be toxic if ingested or inhaled and exposure in children under six has been associated with learning problems, memory loss, and even ADD. Unfortunately, the effects of lead poisoning are irreversible.

Until a massive recall is announced, though, it can be tricky for consumers to know which toys pose a health risk. Recalled toys come in all sizes and shapes and are sold everywhere from independent shops to large chains. What's a parent to do?

Use color as a clue. If the surfaces are painted, check the toy for country of origin, often located on the underside. If the toy was manufactured in China or India, you might reconsider having it in your home.

Don't give kids antique toys. The paint on vintage trucks and dolls is likely to contain lead, since regulations were put into effect only in 1978.

Consult the Consumer Product Safety Commission (CPSC) Web site. The CPSC lists updates of recalled toys. Sign up at cpsc.gov to receive e-mail alerts about future recalls.

Use a lead testing kit. If you're still concerned, buy an inexpensive home-testing kit at a hardware store or online. While these tests are not 100 percent accurate, they may be used as a guide.

Call a doctor. If you believe your child has played with lead-tainted toys or jewelry, call your family physician to request a blood-lead test.

When in doubt, throw it out! As of this writing, many major toy manufacturers and retailers have pledged to strengthen testing standards before toys reach shelves, and Congress has taken up the issue of improving safety oversight. But until we can be assured that our toys are safe, caution is the best policy.

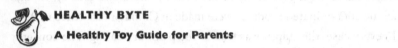

HEALTHY BYTE
A Healthy Toy Guide for Parents

In 2007, The Ecology Center, a Michigan-based nonprofit, came out with a new Web site offering the results of their testing of twelve hundred popular children's toys for toxic chemicals. Parents can search by product name, brand, or toy type to learn how products rate in terms of harmful content. See healthytoys.org.

✺ Expert Opinion ✺
Are *Any* Toys Safe?
By Jennifer Taggart, environmental lawyer, author
of The Smart Mama's Green Guide

All the toys involved in recent recalls—concerning lead in paints and coatings—were made in China. In fact, 80 percent of the world's toys are made in China. How can you make sure your kids' toys are safe?

Safety standards do exist. Under U.S. federal law, the total lead in paints and similar coatings used on toys can't exceed six hundred parts per million (or 0.06 percent). Unfortunately federal law doesn't require that toys actually be checked to assure compliance with this standard before they're sold. Also, the standard is for paint and coatings, not the toy itself. Lead may be present in other components, such as PVC plastic, which is used to make many toys.

There are many "natural" and nontoxic toys on the market. Some manufacturers make bioplastic toys (from corn!). Look for toys that don't use paint or coatings (LEGOs are one example), or that do use plant-based colorants. Online, seek out retailers of "natural toys": While this is not a legal designation, makers of such toys often use plant-based dyes instead of paint; wood (typically sustainable); and textiles that are organic and usually untreated. Where possible, look for the manufacturer's statement on safety/quality (for mid- to large-size toymakers, this may be found on the packaging, but more likely on their Web site; for smaller toymakers, you may not find it at all); how they certify compliance with U.S. standards (random and/or independent testing is good; reliance on suppliers to certify compliance, not so good); and where it was made. Also, look to see if it says "vinyl chloride" or "PVC" on the package. If so, it's best to avoid it.

Parentblog
Prevention Is the Best Medicine
By Noah Wyle, actor

For eleven years, I played an emergency room doctor on TV. During that time, I learned quite a bit about our health-care system. Mostly I learned that it's best to be avoided, if possible. And the smartest way to do that is by taking steps toward leading a healthier life.

Most of the illnesses you see treated in hospitals (with the exception of the ER) are preventable through better diet, more exercise, no smoking, less alcohol, and other lifestyle changes. One of the biggies, as we're just finding out now, is reducing our exposure to toxic chemicals in the environment.

My wife, Tracy, and I were both raised by quasi-hippie parents; our instinct is to do things in a pretty green and natural way. Soon after having kids ourselves, we went through everything in our house to see if we could do better. For instance, we used to clean our bathtub with the most caustic material but didn't really think about the effect of having that toxic residue build up day after day on surfaces that our children come in contact with. Now you'll see Ed Begley's face in most of our cupboards. Baby bottles are another example: My wife was a champion breast-feeder, but occasionally we'd augment with a bottle. Then we found out that if you leave a bottle of water in the car and the temperature of the car heats up, chemicals from the plastic leach into the liquid. It makes perfect rational sense, but why we didn't think of it before I couldn't tell you. Soon we were researching bottles that don't do that, and that's what we now use. In the process of educating ourselves, Tracy became something of a budding toxicologist, and has dragged me to baby expos and health fairs. But her passion has become mine.

Still, you'll drive yourself crazy if you scrutinize every single thing. You have to find a balance between your life and the world around you. Take toys. At the beginning it was easy: We had mostly wooden and other natural toys for the kids to play with—organic stuffed animals, silk scarves, wooden swords. We were so pleased with ourselves. But at birthdays or holidays, well-intentioned friends and family would bring in some plastic or electronic toy, stuff we weren't wild about having in the house. Eventually my son got interested in *Star Wars*, and it's not like they're making wooden action figures. Now we just try to keep things in moderation. We have a good cross-section of toys to play with and everyone's happy.

Then there's food. We try to eat as organically as possible and limit sugar. We're all vegetarians; we're always amazed at people's responses to our kids demanding more salad. But, again, there's a world out there that doesn't always make it feasible to eat healthfully. My children will have cupcakes and candy at birthday parties, and at some point they'll go out and order Big Macs. But if we can start them off with a foundation of health and a philosophy that promotes the benefits of a plant-based diet, then we've done our job.

In the end, living a healthier life is all about balance. But there's a learning curve to it: You have to realize that you can't be perfect, that you just move incrementally toward the optimum choices. Once you start down this path, though, it becomes easier—not to mention more enjoyable, sort of like detective work—to stay on top of the latest information and make new choices to reflect that. And so we keep challenging ourselves to do better. Not too long ago, there was a house that Tracy and I were thinking about buying, a tiny cottage that was so surrounded by nature it was practically off the grid. We described it as the house of the people we *wish* we were. We're diligent and still learning eagerly—but we're not quite there yet.

Step #3. Select Toys That Last

Whether you're buying your child her first dollhouse or you're in plastic-toy rehab after purging a playroom full of PVC, you can really make a statement with the toys you have in your home. As tempted as children are by the diabolical marketing pitches for mass-produced, poorly made products, you can find cool-looking, quality pieces—artisanally made from sustainably grown, organic, and nontoxic materials—that benefit the planet *and* your kids. That way when some giant molded plastic piece does slip in, as it inevitably will, from well-intentioned friends or relatives, you can take it in stride.

Wood is good. Unfinished, solid wood toys are completely healthy for kids, and wood toys with nontoxic paints and finishes release few, if any, harmful chemicals. Natural finishes, like linseed and walnut oil or bees-wax, are beautiful and durable. Solid wood is far preferable to pressed or manufactured woods such as plywood or particle board, which contain glues that can emit fumes.

Look, too, for toys made from recycled wood, which are increasingly available as children's boutiques catch retro-toy fever. Natural toys tend to be pricier than plastic ones, but they're longer lasting and can be kept in the family for years.

Up your healthy fiber quotient. The kind of soft, plush toys that children love to snuggle with are increasingly available in organic, untreated cotton, hemp, and wool and colored with nontoxic dyes. Given that your kid is going to hug and even sleep with her stuffed bunny, you should consider spending the extra for these natural fibers. Conventional stuffed animals and soft-fabric toys may contain flame retardants, dyes, and foam filling. Looking at the bigger picture, cotton production consumes almost a quarter of the world's use of insecticides and 10 percent of its pesticides. Organic fibers, on the other hand, are not treated with chemical fertilizers or pesticides—and wool is a natural flame retardant. Also look for dolls and stuffed animals made from post-consumer recycled materials; the label will no doubt announce this fact.

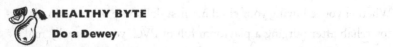

HEALTHY BYTE
Do a Dewey

As in John Dewey, the philosopher and progressive education reformer who believed in "learning by doing" through unstructured exploration. Everyday items make great playthings—they leave more to the imagination and engage the prefrontal cortex, the brain's playroom for abstract thinking: Mixing bowls, utensils, and bakeware, for instance, serve as great stacking toys and noisemakers. (Toddlers love putting shapes into other shapes.) Paper towel rolls, paper bags, and cardboard boxes can be easily decorated and converted into costumes, vehicles, and other role-playing tools. Before recycling old magazines and circulars, help your child cut out favorite pictures and glue them into collages (it develops fine motor skills, too).

For older kids, don't forget the basics: marbles, knitting, woodworking, science experiments, nature exploring. In a technological age, many of these seemingly quaint activities have been abandoned but merit reintroduction. Consult *The Dangerous Book for Boys* by Conn and Hal Iggulden and *The Daring Book for Girls* by Andrea J. Buchanan and Miriam Peskowitz; these wonderful books are packed with imaginative ideas.

Parentblog
Taking Baby Steps
By Anna Getty, environmentalist and columnist
for Yogi Times

The question I like to ask myself is, *How green can I get?* I pose it without getting completely insane about it, but trying to keep it lighthearted and easy. It's about taking baby steps; doing what you can when you can.

I'm always doing research. It makes buying things complicated—I'm on the lookout for what's fair trade, organic, sustainable, or nontoxic. But it also makes me ask myself how badly I need something. I have to admit that sometimes all the searching turns me into a neurotic mess—I've found myself getting down on my husband for not recycling enough—but then I have to remember that he too is learning and taking small steps as well. In the end I don't want to be an eco-elitist. Just a positive example.

Right now we're doing great on the garbage front—our trash guy collects it every two weeks. We've started a compost system. I try to avoid gigantic packaging, and I buy more used and vintage household items. My current project is trying to recycle all the plastic I've collected over the years: baby bottles, toys, sippy cups, etc. I've been going online and searching—I'm convinced there's someone out there who'll take it and recycle it! Meanwhile, I try to bring as little of it into the house as possible. It's a cool challenge to look in the garbage and ask, *How do I make this even less?*

Step #5. Gather a Healthy Layette

For the first few weeks of a baby's life, all she's likely to need is a diaper and undershirt, a swaddling blanket or sleep sack, and maybe some pajamas.

Diaper dos. A baby goes through an average of five to eight thousand diaper changes. No matter which you swear by—cloth or disposable— your decision has far-reaching consequences. Disposables are made of paper, plastic, and absorptive gel. Mostly nonbiodegradable, they leave heaps of plastic in landfills for decades—3.6 million tons per year, according to EPA estimates. Obviously it's a scourge on the environment, but are disposable diapers unhealthy for babies, too?

Disposables contain chemicals that were banned in the 1980s in women's tampons, but continue to be used to improve absorbency. They can also emit gases like toluene, xylene, and styrene, and since babies inhale more air per pound of body weight than adults do and are generally more affected by the toxicity of air pollutants, this is troubling. There are really very few studies on how chemicals in diapers might affect baby's health, but as with any chemical exposure, it's better to be cautious.

Cloth diapers are a time-tested green option and many diaper services have emerged in recent years. But for many parents the cloth route is a bit challenging—they're tricky to secure and a hassle to wash, and can pose a drain on energy and water. (Then again, they can be reused dozens of times, lowering their eco-impact.)

Fortunately there are now several nonchlorinated, more biodegradable disposable diaper brands available. There's also gDiapers, consisting of eco-safe disposable diaper liners in reusable pants. Many parents improvise with some combination of cloth and disposable diapers; experiment until you find what makes you and your child most comfortable.

Parentblog
Change a Diaper, Change the World
By Jason and Kim Graham-Nye, cofounders of gDiapers

One day over breakfast, my wife Kim and I came across an amazing statistic: Every day 50 million disposable diapers enter landfills in America. Wow, we thought, that is a lot of plastic and poop! We continued to learn that each diaper takes up to five hundred years to biodegrade. We were shocked. We were about to have our first child and couldn't imagine joining the landfill train. The only problem was, we were in drought-stricken

Australia where water is more valuable than gold, which meant cloth diapers also had their environmental downside. When our son was four months old, we found an earth-friendly diaper option made by a Tasmanian company. They were flushable and compostable, so they didn't have to end up in the landfill. We couldn't believe how empowering it was to use them, and with ten or so diaper changes a day, we got to feel good over and over again.

For us, the simple act of changing our son's diapers truly changed our lives. Not that we didn't care about the earth before, but it just got a whole lot more personal. We paid more attention to how things were made, how they would affect his tiny body, and how they impacted the planet. With diapers, this is all particularly relevant because your baby is in them 24/7. The new diapers we found were breathable and thus more comfortable. The flushables didn't contain plastic, which meant they were better environmentally and certainly better for our son. They were even certified "Cradle to Cradle," which meant they would be no burden on the earth, plus they would be reabsorbed back into the ecosystem in a neutral or beneficial way. We thought this was all pretty cool.

As it turns out, there are a lot of other parents who think so too. We ended up buying the rights to the technology and moved our family halfway around the world to launch gDiapers in America. We weren't environmentalists looking for a business—simply parents in search of a better way to cover our baby's bottom.

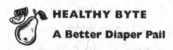

HEALTHY BYTE
A Better Diaper Pail

Those fancy diaper systems, meant to lock each soiled nappy in its own section of plastic, sound good in theory (thirty diapers . . . hermetically sealed!). In reality, these pails begin to stink pretty quickly, and the plastic they're made of, not to mention the bags, contain unwanted chemicals. Do yourself and your baby a favor: Put diapers in the regular trash.

Or keep a tight-lidded, small metal can near the changing table and clean it out daily, emptying any "firm" contents into the toilet before throwing away. And wash your hands when you're done!

Swaddling blanket. For at least the first three months of life, an infant is comforted by the feeling of being wrapped in a tight little bundle, just as he was in the womb. Healthy Child advisor Dr. Harvey Karp, author and creator of the book/DVD *The Happiest Baby on the Block*, refers to this stage as the "fourth trimester." Although babies are routinely swaddled in hospital nurseries, many parents stop this practice soon after they get home, unaware that babies miss the protective envelopment of the womb and are upset by their own flailing limbs. This makes a large, square receiving blanket a great addition to your layette, and parents can now find brands of baby wraps that close with velcro to simplify the technique. If you can, pick an organic cotton one.

Little essentials. A newborn's layette typically consists of a few cotton onesies, side-snap undershirts, receiving blankets, leggings, towels, pajamas, socks, and booties. All should ideally be in untreated, certified organic cotton: Babies' skin is extra-sensitive, so the purer the fabric, the better.

Parentblog
Developing Thicker Skin
By Paige Goldberg Tolmach, owner of The Little Seed

My son, Jackson, developed extreme eczema within the first eight weeks of life. His doctors told me that his skin condition was a product of genetics and a reaction to the weather. This seemed odd to me, as neither my husband nor I had eczema. They wanted to treat him with topical and oral steroids and said if we were lucky, he might grow out of it by age six.

This wasn't good enough for me. In my heart, I knew that they were wrong. I kept on searching for answers. I did a tremendous amount of research on eczema, allergies, and possible dietary and environmental factors that might have played a role. What I discovered was shocking. I had no idea that so many things in my home contained sensitizing and even toxic ingredients. Within days I was dumping the crib mattress and plastic toys and chemical-based cleansers; I bought organic clothing and sheets and opened windows all over the house. And sure enough, as soon as I got rid of many of the chemicals in Jackson's immediate environment, his skin started to clear up.

I wanted to get up on the rooftops and start shouting. Here I was, a pretty smart, well-educated person who just didn't know *any* of this. And if I didn't, it stood to reason that a lot of other parents didn't either. I was so relieved to have found a way to help my baby, but I was angry too that this information was so hard to find.

Lacking a plan for what to do next, I improvised. I noticed that when I put Jackson into the car seat, for example, he would develop welts all over his arm. So I made him a car seat cover out of organic fabric. I searched the globe for healthy, organic toys for him. I ordered an all-natural willow rattle from New Zealand, nontoxic wooden trucks from Arkansas, and vegetable-dyed soft toys from Sri Lanka. Although I was determined to find these safer, cleaner things for him, I kept thinking that it shouldn't be so hard. Parents should be better informed and they should have options. That's where I got the idea to create a store where all of these things—organic clothing, low-VOC-emitting cribs, nontoxic crayons—would exist under one roof.

It's been hard, but I feel like my eyes are open for the first time in my life, and my baby did this for me. We think that we have so much to teach them in this world when, in actuality, they are really teaching us. It's a wonderful realization to make. And it's the most beautiful thing in the world.

Step #6. Clothes Call

Kids outgrow clothes faster than a parent can keep up (you know that high-water pants look). As with toys, the best solution—for earth and wallet both—is to tap a flowing spigot of hand-me-downs, whether through family and friends or consignment shops or tag sales. The clothes will seem new to your kid, even if they're gently worn, and any chemicals used in the manufacturing process will have been eliminated by repeated washings. Indeed, synthetic fabric finishes are frequently applied to polyester and polyester-blend clothing (you can tell it's there from the chemical smell and slippery feel of the material).

Don't dress your little sheep in wolf's clothing: Organic clothing is healthy for your kids and less taxing to the earth, too. The toxic residue from the pesticides and herbicides used in conventional cotton crop production pollutes the soil and waterways. Organic wool—from sheep raised without synthetic hormones and without chemical treatments—is available in abundance, as are fabrics made of bamboo, hemp, and flax, though these tend to be a bit pricier than many conventionally made duds. (Fortunately you can find these online, in many children's boutiques, in catalogs, and increasingly at big chain stores like Wal-Mart, Garnet Hill, and Pottery Barn.) But here's what you're buying: all-natural materials that require no toxic chemicals to grow or fabricate. If organic clothing is too pricey, consider splurging at least on organic pajamas, given the amount of time kids spend in them. The pj's should indicate whether they meet the federal safety requirement for sleepwear (which for most untreated, natural-material jammies means they must be snug-fitting).

Still, it's pretty hard to avoid conventional baby clothes, which are cheaper and far more widely available. Prewash all new purchases, but skip those synthetic-perfumed laundry soaps marketed as "baby safe" and opt instead for eco-friendly detergent that contains all-natural ingredients with no chlorine bleach.

Step #7. Be a Smart Gearhead

In our vigilance to be armed and ready for parenthood, we tend to buy more gear than we need—electric bottle warmers, baby gyms, kid corrals. How did our parents ever survive without them? Quite easily. Are most of them necessary? Of course not. Before buying, investigate consumer feedback on consumer Web sites or ask around to see whether or not others got any use out of them.

From a health standpoint, the goal is to avoid bringing unnecessary plastic and foam containing plasticizers, flame retardants, and heavy metals into your home. I've broken my nose three times, so it was Jessica who had to point out to me that the new infant car seat I'd just pulled out of the box had a strong chemical smell. If a piece of equipment is too malodorous, put it on the porch or in the garage to air it out for a day or even longer, if possible. After a week, I brought our seat inside. "Now?" I asked. "Still stinks," she said. One week later, it finally passed the sniff test.

High chairs. Like all children's gear, high chairs are regulated by the Consumer Product Safety Commission; if you're in the market for one, you can find recall information on the CPSC site (cpsc.gov). Another good resource is *Consumer Reports*, which tests kids' gear for safety (consumerreports.org). One other thing to keep in mind: Some foam-padded high chairs may contain polyurethane foam in the cushion. You can find beautiful, durable wooden high chairs with natural cushions on many green design and children's gear Web sites (see Healthy Resources); some even convert to chairs that can be lowered and pulled up to the table once your toddler outgrows them.

Car seats. In 2007, a Michigan environmental group named Ecology Center released a study indicating that unwanted chemicals like chlorine, bromine, and lead could be leaching from car seats. Of the sixty-two car seat models they tested, 30 percent had elevated levels of the chemicals; the two biggest culprits were PVCs and flame retardants. (Those free of the chemicals included the Graco SnugRide [Emerson] and EvenFlo Discovery-Churchill infant seats.) For a list of the best and worst seats, check out healthycar.org. No matter which car seat model you buy, however, air it out for a few days in your yard or other outdoor space.

Saucer entertainers and swings. These items provide great baby distraction when you need to cook or do any task requiring arms. In other words, they've become pretty indispensable. They may also be stimulating, in a good way. I'm not suggesting you carry your baby at all times—though baby carrying is experiencing a renaissance among modern parents, who've read of the calming effect to babies of the constant jiggling and warmth of being snuggled up against a parent's chest or back. But think hard before making this purchase. For one, both types of items are made of huge pieces of molded plastic, which as you know can release fumes for a while after they're out of the box. Also, your baby will be able to suck and even chew on some of the attached plastic toys. Perhaps the best compromise is to get a used one. And to pay it forward when you're done by reselling, donating, or Freecycling it.

Cribs and mattresses. Nearly all conventional baby mattresses today use materials that contain unwanted and potentially harmful ingredients like flame retardants and formaldehyde. If you can, opt for an organic mattress, made of cotton or wool or both, and consider a naturally finished wood crib. Read all about these healthy options in Chapter 9.

Step #8. Use Greener Art Supplies

Art and hobby products, even those aimed at young kids, can contain hidden health hazards, such as lead in ceramic glazes and solvents in glues. Companies are not required by law to list toxic ingredients, only whether the products contain serious hazards along the lines of "fatal if swallowed."

To reassure consumers, many art supply makers have sought certification by the nonprofit Art and Creative Materials Institute (ACMI) and have voluntarily agreed to have their materials evaluated by independent toxicologists for safety. The ACMI grants its Approved Product (AP) label if a product contains no hazardous ingredients. If a product does contain toxic chemicals, it gets a CL or Cautionary Label. It's not fail-safe (see the crayon incident, below), but until parents and other consumers demand more complete disclosure of harmful ingredients from all manufacturers, it's the best benchmark we have.

Read labels. For young children, pick products that carry ACMI's AP label and avoid those that warn against use by grade six and under. California's Environmental Health Office has a list of supplies not allowed for use in grades K-6 that can serve as a guideline (go to oehha.org and search "art hazards list"). Also seek out products labeled "low odor"; many art supplies, including markers, pens, and paint thinners, are now formulated to produce fewer fumes. And if a product says "danger," "warning," "caution," or "harmful or fatal if swallowed"—well, that's a pretty obvious sign to steer clear.

If you're still concerned about the chemicals in a given art product, ask the manufacturer for its Material Safety Data Sheet (MSDS), which lists ingredients and potential health hazards.

Get little artists to scrub up. Young kids put things in their mouths, accidentally and not. When they finish their masterworks, they should wash hands and brushes well.

Crayons and chalk. After the *Seattle Post-Intelligencer* published an investigative study in 2000 that turned up asbestos in Crayola, Prang, and Rose Art crayons—all of which carried the AP safety label—the offending substance was removed. (Asbestos isn't an ingredient but a contaminant of talc, which was used as a crayon strengthener.) Most crayons are petroleum-based but you can also buy soybean and beeswax crayons, too. And check out "no dust" chalk online or at office supply stores.

Good glues. Stick to glues less likely to emit VOC fumes. Rubber cement, which you probably played with as a kid, is particularly nasty: It contains hexane, a neurotoxin. Elmer's glue is much safer than many other glues; in stick form it's even better because it's less likely to get on skin or be inhaled. Mucilage and white library paste are also fine. Natural school glues can be found at green supply stores online.

Clean clays. Polymer clays are labeled as nontoxic by ACMI, yet they're made of PVCs softened with phthalates. (ACMI argues that the amount is too small to cause harm.) Concerned parents can find safer clays made of beeswax or natural play dough at green art supply stores. (See Healthy Resources at the back of the book.)

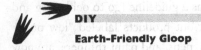

DIY
Earth-Friendly Gloop

Kids love to squeeze this oozy, blobby version of play dough through their fingers. Have them wear smocks and work in an easy-to-clean area.

a few drops natural food or juice coloring (see seelecttea.com or recipe below)

1 cup water

1 cup cornstarch

Add food coloring to water and mix with cornstarch in a bowl. Children can then squeeze and prod the gloop. Store in a covered container; revive periodically from drying out with a bit of water.

Kid-safe paints. Stick with watercolor and (water-based) tempura paints, which don't contain dangerous solvents that give off VOCs. Teens who want to work in oil paint should use water-soluble oils; look for those bearing the AP label. To clean brushes, try swishing them in baby oil followed by soap and rinse with water rather than turpentine.

Pens and markers. Opt for "low odor" markers instead of stinky ones, which may contain potent solvents. In particular, writing tools labeled "permanent" or "waterproof" emit higher levels of airborne, easily inhaled particles. For white board dry-erase markers, again choose the low-odor kind. And bypass scented markers, which expose children to synthetic fragrances to sniff, or even taste.

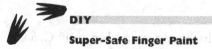

DIY

Super-Safe Finger Paint

⅓ cup soap flakes melted with ½ cup boiling water
1 cup cornstarch
⅓ cup cold water
a few drops juice dyes (see below)

Make your own soap flakes by grating a bar of homemade hand soap (available in your health food store) until you have ⅓ cup of it. Combine the cornstarch, cold water, and melted soap in a bowl. Stir to blend. Let the mixture set until it's thick. Divide into separate bowls and stir in juice dyes.

Homemade juice dyes. These can be used for everything from dyeing paper to coloring homemade finger paints, plus they're pretty fun. Play around with different bright foods to see what works, including blueberries and red onion skins (purple), cranberries and beets (red), turmeric (yellow), or paprika and coffee (brown). Combine a quarter cup of the food with two cups water; simmer over low heat for an hour. Cool, strain, and use. Add to finger paints or your play dough.

Step #9. Green Your Student

Since kids can spend six hours a day (or more) at school, make sure they go chemical-free when on the move. See Healthy Resources for recommended products and brands.

Reuse first. Kids beg for new backpacks, lunch boxes, and notebooks at the start of each school year. While the back-to-school shopping ritual is exciting, if you've got adequate supplies and your child's gear is still in good shape, try to reuse at least some of what you've got and recycle everything you can.

Carry a better backpack. Many backpacks are made with PVC, a.k.a. vinyl. You can avoid it by purchasing brands made of nylon or polyester; you can also find backpacks made of durable recycled materials online. Reused canvas and leather bags are also good options.

Find greener school supplies. Hunt for products that are recycled/ recyclable and chemical-free. For paper, look for processed chlorine free (PCF) or totally chlorine free (TCF) brands made with the highest percentage of postconsumer recycled content possible. Teach your children to reuse single-sided sheets or use both sides of the notebook page. You can find recycled binders and notebooks at green office supply stores and even many mainstream purveyors. For guidelines on art supplies and glues that don't give off VOC fumes, see Step #8.

Get the lead out of the lunch box. Most lunch boxes are made of vinyl and, according to a 2007 study by the consumer watchdog group Center for Environmental Health, many contain undesirable levels of lead. Since the report, many manufacturers have taken steps to improve their testing and reporting; look for a LEAD FREE label. Better yet, use a reusable cloth sack or a metal or recycled-material lunch box.

Step #10. Tone Down the Electronics

So many kids' toys speak, flash, blurt, sing, and move on battery power. (What parent doesn't know the frustration of trying to locate the monkey that won't stop yapping from somewhere deep in the toy chest?) Even babies are now spectators of a constant sound and light show from their toys and gear. Manufacturers may argue that such games stimulate and educate, but the argument is largely, well, manufactured: Simpler is usually better—for pedagogical reasons as well as human and ecological health.

3 billion average number of batteries Americans buy each year for radios, cell phones, watches, toys, laptop computers, and portable power tools.
(Environmental Protection Agency, 2006)

Electronics are also inevitably made from plastic and run on batteries that pose their own problems: They can leak toxic acids that burn little hands; and when they end up in the landfill, they leach pollutants into soil and groundwater. If you go electronic, choose rechargeable, recyclable batteries—or toys that use solar power. The Rechargeable Battery Recycling Corporation has collection sites throughout the country (see rbrc. org).

A note about computers: These days kids are logging on before they can tie their own shoes. Many computers are treated with flame retardants, so if you're buying new, look for one that adheres to the EPA's Electronic Product Environmental Assessment Tool (EPEAT), which is based on European standards for fifty-one environmental criteria including restrictions on cadmium, lead, mercury, and flame retardants.

 ONE STEP BEYOND

Start a toy and book swap club. Get together with other parents for an exchange party. Most kids really don't care if a toy is used; they're just excited to have something different. However, you'll want to be discerning about inviting people that share your parenting philosophy so you don't end up with PVC toys, play guns, or something else you may not want in your home.

Demand safer toys. Call retailers like Toys "R" Us (800-869-7787) to stop carrying PVC products; call toy manufacturers like Hasbro/Play-skool (hasbro.com, 800-242-7276), Mattel (800-524-8697), and Fisher-Price (800-432-5437) to stop making them.

CHAPTER 6

Splendor in the Grass

GREENER GARDENS, YARDS,
AND OUTDOOR SPACES

When I was a child growing up in Connecticut, we lived by a pristine New England stream. My three brothers and I spent countless hours exploring in and around "the river": climbing over boulders, swimming, rock skipping, fishing for sparkling brook and rainbow trout, clearing it of fallen tree limbs. We felt as if we were its caretakers. This was our space, our haven.

One summer, my father called a local lawn maintenance company to fertilize our front yard, which abutted the stream. I remember men with big green hoses spraying the yard with torrents of chemical fertilizers and weed killers. Four days later, the lawn was as green as a pool table. But when my brothers and I went down to the water, like we'd done hundreds of times, the brook was littered with dead trout.

"What happened?" I asked.

When my father came down, he looked perplexed. "They must be sick," he said.

"It's the chemicals," said my brother. My father shook his head in disbelief.

I think it's fair to call this a formative memory.

I don't tell this story to portray my father, who enjoys the outdoors, as callous or clueless: That's what suburban homeowners did back then, before they knew the consequences. Unfortunately, maintaining a velvety lawn is still something of a national obsession, and many homeowners continue to use such chemicals to create what is literally a supernatural carpet of grass. Every year, more than 90 million pounds of pesticides are showered on American lawns; we use seven to ten times more pesticides per acre of lawn than farmers use on food crops. Doing so regularly may make your grounds look like a movie set. That's the short run.

Synthetic fertilizers and pesticides strike far deeper than those three inches of green. What lies beneath that thin layer of grass isn't just dirt but a thriving world of insects, worms, microbes, fungi, and nutrients that are thrown into turmoil and can be wiped out quickly by the application of these chemicals—chemicals that, ironically, can make the grass *more* susceptible to disease. Besides, in time, the very plants and insects being tamed by these chemicals adapt to them, hence the development and application of *new* potent concoctions. Then there's the picture beyond the lawn: the long-term pollution of air and water, and their potential impact on the health of our families and pets.

Simply put: Organic gardening allows us to avoid using harmful chemical sprays and powders on our plants. But it goes way beyond that. It recognizes the deeper truth that a garden is a complete universe of plants, water, insects, and wildlife kept in perfect balance through acts of nature. Anyone who loves gardening knows it's a constant, delicate push-pull between control and chaos, coaxing certain plants to thrive while keeping others from overtaking. Organic gardening begins with the soil, incorporates natural defenses against pests and weeds, results in a beautiful and diverse landscape, and ends once more with healthy, vital soil.

50 percentage of total lifetime pesticide exposure that occurs during the first five years of one's life. (National Academy of Sciences, 1993)

We want our children to love the feeling of digging in the dirt with their hands, of playing outdoors and in field sports, of discovering nature in ways that enhance, rather than jeopardize, their health. Here are ways to make your family's outdoor space more beautiful and cleaner—so your kids can get dirty safely.

Step #1. Green Your Lawn

Kids love to roll around on grass, throw handfuls at each other (to the dismay of the family lawn tender), maybe chew on a blade. But most lawns subsist on a brew of chemical fertilizers and herbicides, which don't exactly stay put—they come off on skin and clothing. In fact, children aged six to eleven have been found to possess higher levels of lawn chemicals in their blood than adults, according to the CDC, studies show cancer in children (and pets) is elevated in relation to the amounts of pesticides and herbicides used on lawns and gardens, among other places.

It's easy to maintain a lawn without using all this plant "junk food" by following green principles. The results won't come overnight, as they seem to with chemical products, but they *will* come, and you'll have the satisfaction of knowing two things: organic gardening is better for grass; and it's much safer for the children and pets who use it. Another thing: Over the long term, keeping up with yard work will be a whole lot easier for you than for your tank-and-hose-touting neighbor.

Get in the zone. Ask your local nursery which grasses are native to your area. Indigenous grasses work with the conditions in your yard, and will be easier to cultivate—meaning less fertilizer, pesticides, water, and maintenance. Keep in mind that blade grass needs about six hours of sun a day; if your yard gets less, consider bringing in other types of easy-to-grow, shade-loving ground cover—on short grades or near the house—or create scattered perennial gardens to reduce the lawn surface area you must manage. Besides, keeping a variety of plants, both grasses and flowering plants, draws beneficial insects and looks beautiful.

Mow high. Tall grass absorbs more light and water and shades out weeds. Set your mower blade to two to three inches from the ground and never take off more than the top one-third of the blade (and don't mow when the grass is wet). If you leave your clippings on the lawn, they can recycle nitrogen back into the soil (a natural, free fertilizer!). Rake away clumps of leaves, though.

Aerate often. Compacted soil is bad for grass—the roots need air and water to penetrate the soil. Rent a small aerator machine from your local nursery or, with your kids, stomp around on the lawn in spiked shoes (golf cleats or shoe attachments are available at garden supply stores). The best aerator? The earthworm, which thrives in pesticide-free soil, and will take up residence in your grass if you don't douse it with chemicals.

Keep your soil fit. Maintain neutral pH levels in your soil and use organic phosphate-free fertilizers or compost to build nutrients in the dirt. Organic fertilizers, available at garden supply stores, release their nutrients slowly and pose no threat to beneficial organisms. (For more on fertilizing, see Step #4.)

 HEALTHY BYTE
Say It Loud—Pesticide-Free and Proud!

Declare your yard free of toxic chemicals by posting a PESTICIDE FREE sign. (The signs are also handy for schools and businesses.) Order a small lawn sign for seven dollars from the Washington Toxics Coalition (watoxics.org, 800-844-SAFE).

Water truly, deeply, infrequently. Lawns are the single most irrigated crop in the United States, according to NASA—about 40 million acres in total. Fortunately, despite what chronic lawn fretters think, grass needs only about an inch of water a week. Water early—5 to 8 A.M. is best—and deeply (light spritzing weakens roots). Overwatering can create fungus, so let the grass dry out before resprinkling. Be attentive to your seasonal and regional rainfall: If you get a healthy shower (keep a container outside to measure how much), then don't water that week.

Spread your seed. Grass grows best when nights are cool, so fall is the best time to reseed and fill in bare spots. Also, unless you're severely allergic to bees, add a little clover to your grass mix; it's drought- and disease-resistant.

Parentblog
My Big Fat Greek Garden
By Melina Kanakaredes, actress

Growing up in Akron, Ohio, right in front of a state park, I definitely had an appreciation for nature—playing outside until dark, the streetlights signaling it was time to come in, was one of the formative memories of my youth. But that deep connection to nature came principally from spending summers in Greece with my grandparents, who were born there, and my extended family. Everyone in our village had a garden, and on Fridays we would pick our own grape leaves and eat them stuffed. I'd swim in the ocean and pull mussels off the rocks, which we'd cook for dinner that night. I'd bring buckets to the man with the cow for milk, and of course we always had locally made olive oil. My parents referred to our diet as "peasant food," but it was delicious and fresh. I never once heard the word "organic," but we lived it. It just makes so much sense to live off of the bounty of everything around you—for food as well as for other basic human ministrations. Because of my cultural background, a lot of products I used contained natural ingredients—olive oil–based shampoos and soaps. As a Greek kid, that was your medicine. You fell and hurt yourself? Put olive oil on the bruise. I may have smelled like salad but the bruises went away quickly.

When you become a parent, you're offered a chance to do things in a new way, to be more conscious about the decisions you make because each one affects more than just you. You want to give your children the greatest parts of what your parents gave you and then maybe take it even a step further. From my family I learned a respect for using and not abusing the land, not taking it for granted. Now I'm trying to convey to my two girls the value in simple things, especially given the opulence of LA and big-city life: eating fresh food from the farmers' market; looking for fairies or lightning bugs in the woods rather than sitting in front of the TV; observing how the flowers and trees change with the seasons.

We love watching things grow. In our yard we have some amazing fruit trees—grapefruit, lemon, fig—which remind me so much of Greece. You can just grab the grapefruit off the tree and eat it for breakfast. I'm always yanking figs off our tree for a snack. My father-in-law, who's also Greek, likes to pull a cucumber out of the garden when he gets to the house and eat it with sea salt. Just as in Greece, where everything's natural, we don't use pesticides. I can't contemplate putting poison on all this incredible greenery, not to mention in places where my girls play. I've only started to dabble in organic gardening—my husband is the maestro at it, but I keep up the effort to assist—and being the granddaughter of immigrants, it's ingrained in me not to waste anything. To me, respect for the environment is simply another core value we can give our children, like respect for family or good manners. It's something I work on doing a little bit, every day. Because it's really our contribution not just to them but to *their* children.

Step #2. Whack Weeds Without Herbicides

In the battle of man versus nature, learning to live with a few weeds is the gardener's mark of maturity. Still, weeds compete with your carefully coaxed plants for water, nutrients, sunlight, and growing space, and should be thinned for more than just aesthetic reasons. Here are some eco-friendly tips for taming:

Yank them young (and teach your young to yank them). Your first defense against weeds: Pull or hoe them before they become established and their roots plunge deep into the soil. All you really need is fifteen minutes a week to keep up with new growth. If you're not sure what's a weed and what isn't, let the plant grow a while and see how you like it. It's a relative term, anyway: One person's weed is another person's ivy patch.

Recruit your kids to weed, too. A few handfuls of weeds in a bucket of water can make a convincing "magic potion." (Adding imagination to the exercise can inspire a child to become a compulsive weeder.)

Mulch ado. Cover your garden soil once a season with mulch to block weeds. Without adequate light, weeds can't produce enough chlorophyll to grow. Mulch also conserves water, keeps roots cool, and nourishes the soil as it decomposes.

Organic mulches include a wide range of materials such as compost, wood chips, shredded bark, hay, cocoa bean shells, grass clippings, shredded leaves, peat moss, or brown bags, straw, and other biodegradable materials. Avoid all tire mulch and the red-dyed type of wood mulch, which is typically made from mixed hardwoods and wood waste that may contain an arsenic-laced preservative called chromated copper arsenate (CCA); it's then dyed red to cover the impurities in the wood. (Not all red mulches contain CCA, though, so check the label or contact the manufacturer if you like the look.)

A two- to three-inch layer of mulch keeps sunlight from tickling the weed seeds, thereby thwarting their germination. Apply early in the growing season, just after weeding or digging your soil. Take care to leave a two-inch radius around plant stems to prevent root rot from moisture trapped in the mulch.

Kill them softly. With patience, you can eliminate weeds the natural way. One reliable weapon is a natural corn-gluten herbicide such as WeedBan, available at green garden supply stores, which is safe for kids and pets (though don't apply it when you're seeding new grass or you'll knock out the grass, too). The acid-based herbicides certified for organic growing are, not surprisingly, less powerful than glyphosate, the active ingredient in Roundup, but over time are just as effective.

Or try a homegrown herbicide. You can pickle weeds by pouring distilled white vinegar into a spray bottle and evenly coating them with it. Vinegar is 5 percent acetic acid, which burns the plant, especially on sunny days. Take care not to douse your favorite garden plants, though, as the vinegar can kill them, too. Or you can just pour boiling water over problem plants, which kills both weed seeds and the living leaf. Okay, so maybe it's not such a soft way to go after all.

Hoe down. Annual weeds die when you cut the stems from the roots just below the soil, easily accomplished with a sharp hoe. An ordinary garden hoe will do, or get your hands on a swan-neck hoe, which is easier for your back. If you have an infestation of dandelions, get specific weeding tools, such as the Weed Hound or Dandelion Terminator, at gardening stores. But try to embrace some of these flowers. Kids love dandelions, so keep a few for making crowns.

Step #3. Enrich Your Soil

Organic gardeners are obsessed with making superior soil. The process is part science and part art, as you replenish nutrients to keep the earth vital, and mix organic matter into it to speed the nourishing decomposition of nature. Such efforts can yield rich, dark, loamy soil popping with life-giving earthworms, the best fertility builder you can find.

Test your soil. To create a healthy garden or lawn, you first need to know what your dirt is made of. There are three elements in soil: sand, clay, and silt. Ideally you want an equal balance of each, yielding a neutral pH. You can get a soil test for about ten dollars through your county's cooperative extension offices (csrees.usda.gov/extension). The test tells you the soil's pH and which nutrients are out of balance. You can also buy test kits in stores or online. Once you know your lawn's strengths and weaknesses, add the appropriate elements to adjust. If your soil is too acidic, compensate with lime; if too alkaline, balance it with pine needles, peat moss, or wood ashes. The key is to tend to it like you're cooking a stew: a pinch of this, a dash of that—*magnifique*.

Go compost crazy. Compost comes from decomposing organic matter (grass clippings, leaves, branches, and fruit and vegetable scraps). It looks like rich, black silt, and when it's spread around the garden, it releases nutrients gradually. Unlike synthetic fertilizers, which give plants a jolt of growth factor and then acidify the soil—essentially killing off its most vital elements—compost *feeds* organisms that are key components of soil building. It keeps the soil aerated, holds water, and decreases your trash loads.

Compost can be made at home, for those dedicated enough to save their kitchen and garden scraps and turn the compost bin regularly, which encourages air circulation and decomposition. (See "One Step Beyond: Build a Worm Farm with Your Kids" at the end of this chapter.) You can also buy ready-to-use compost at any big gardening or home supply store.

Rotate crops. Old-fashioned crop rotation helps keep the soil rich in nutrients. When you plant the same thing in the same location year after year, it's likely to yield increasingly anemic harvests because the soil becomes depleted of nitrogen. This is the "art part" of gardening: Each year you can create some variety, so the garden is always transforming into something new to behold.

 ## Parentblog

Naked . . . in New York?

By Keri Russell, actress

Last summer I was sitting with a couple of friends, watching our naked babies on the grass. We were in Martha's Vineyard, where my husband was raised; my son, River, and the others, all born within three months of each other, were lying and rolling around without diapers, occasionally peeing on the lawn and happily flapping their little arms and legs.

It made me think about how, when a baby is born, their skin is so clean and so pure (I know that's a lame term, but it's true!). But then we wash them in all these soaps and perfumed shampoos, slather on cream, clean them with wipes and put them in these tight, often plastic diapers. On some level, it just doesn't make sense. A baby's skin should take care of itself. Laundry is another thing. I didn't think you had to be so stringent about what you wash your baby's clothes in, but one time I ran out of eco-safe detergent and washed one of River's blankets in the regular stuff. Later, his skin broke out in a rash. Their bodies are so small and sensitive, it's kind of eye-opening in the way it makes you realize just how exposed we are to so many toxic chemicals in the environment.

My friends and I were saying that we wish our babies could always just run around without clothes and that we wouldn't have to worry about what's in the grass, or about other kinds of outdoor pollution. But we live in New York City, which makes such carefree parenting impossible. Still, if you try hard enough, I think you can find a little bit of nature anywhere. On the Vineyard, everyone goes to the farmers' market and talks to the farmers and their neighbors—it's like getting news from the big city; I love how old-fashioned it feels. But I do the same in Brooklyn, where my local farmers' market in summers is piled high with corn, rhubarb, blueberries, strawberries, raspberries, and all those beautiful green vegetables. It's great knowing that most of the food is organic, but more than that, it's so cool to talk to the guys selling milk—getting my news from the country! On the Vineyard you pay to get your garbage taken off the island, so everyone composts their own waste. It makes people inventive in a way that I've definitely brought back to the city, where (in Brooklyn, at least) you're responsible for taking out your trash. Next year I'm planning to start a garden in back of our brownstone. I hope we'll be able to grow tomatoes or peas or something else we can eat. Still, I'm hardly perfect on the healthy living front. I'm still learning. You can't make yourself crazy—well, some people can, some people have all day long just to be healthy, and that's great for them. But what's nice is that there's so much information out there now on how to make better choices, it's much easier to do all this stuff.

Recently I took River for a walk in Fort Greene Park early in the morning, when the park is at its prettiest and all the dogs are out and off the leash.

There are always families with strollers and babies toddling around this little green oasis. If you squint your eyes you wouldn't know you were in New York City. And I can't help but think that if we keep cleaning up our act, maybe someday our babies will be able to roll around naked on the grass here, too.

Step #4. Fertilize Naturally

You may not need to fertilize, period, if you keep your soil enriched, eschew chemical pesticides, and otherwise keep your plants healthy. But if you do need to give your garden a little boost, look for organic fertilizers made from vegetable, animal, and mineral sources. From your soil test (described in the previous step), you'll know whether your garden or lawn lacks nitrogen, phosphorous, or potassium (N, P, or K respectively). Commercially available fertilizer is marked with three numbers representing the amount of each of these nutrients (called the "NPK ratio"). You can balance your deficiency with the appropriate naturally derived source; most of the following are generally available at gardening or home improvement stores. Sources of organic fertilizer include:

Nitrogen (N): Blood meal, alfalfa meal, coffee grounds, cottonseed meal, compost, grass clippings, eggshells, fish emulsion, feathers, hair, ground lobster shells.

Phosphorous (P): Compost, rock phosphate, ground coconut shells, ground oyster shells.

Potassium (K): Potash rock, fireplace wood ash, kelp, soybean meal, granite dust, green sand.

Fertilize in the fall and in midspring. You won't see results immediately as you do with chemical products—the soil's organisms take time to digest the nutrients—but you'll reap the benefits over time.

Step #5. Kick the Chemical Pesticide Habit

Sure, conventional pesticides kill unwanted bugs, but they also do much more than that: They attack friendly, helpful bugs; they don't always kill the bugs you target; and over time they contribute to the evolution of stronger bugs that resist these poisons. Moreover, they can be transferred by a phenomenon known as "pesticide drift" into our homes, which puts the whole family at risk of exposure. Most insecticides work by attacking the nervous systems of bugs and other species, including—potentially—humans. Some studies have suggested a link between excessive pesticide exposure and childhood leukemia; others point to interference with immune and endocrine systems. Grim news for all, but especially for kids and pregnant women, who should be especially wary of chemical pesticide exposure as it may contribute to birth defects.

10

Number of times *indoor* **pesticide levels can increase after an** *outdoor* **application.**

(Environmental Health Perspectives, 2001)

Clearly, the old "spray and pray" method is no longer an option. Sure, all gardens have pests—but an infestation means that its ecosystem is out of whack: too much or too little water, an imbalance of nutrients, or other factors impervious to pesticides. The key to reducing pests is to maintain a healthy garden or lawn by using organic methods that preserve harmony among your garden's various natural checks and balances.

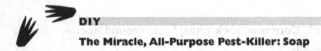

DIY

The Miracle, All-Purpose Pest-Killer: Soap

How does soap kill pests? It dehydrates them.

Mix one to two tablespoons liquid Castile soap with one gallon water. Spray infested areas. Watch bugs slide off.

Recruit your own bug army. Make your garden a place where nature, especially bugs, can help keep pests in check. For example, ladybugs, which you can find at nurseries or garden centers, like to eat aphids, while lacewings chow down on moth eggs and caterpillars. Lure these beneficial bugs by growing small plants with accessible nectar, like lovage, dill, fennel, and sweet alyssum. (All of these helpful predators go running in search of food when they encounter heavy-duty pesticides, another reason to curb their use.) Let spiders take up residence in your woodpile or shed, and hang a bird feeder or two.

Practice "companion planting." A diversely laid out garden minimizes damage to entire sections, and growing vegetables beside plants with different odors and root secretions helps to divert pests. For example, marigolds emit an odor that bugs don't like; sweet basil repels aphids, mites, and mosquitoes, and acts as a fungicide. (For more information on companion planting and happy plant couples, see the helpful site seedsofchange.com.)

 BURNING QUESTION
What's the best natural way to fend off mosquitoes?

DEET has long been hailed as the most potent spray-on insect repellent, but the chemical can have side effects, especially on kids. Here are ways to get mosquitoes to bug off without overusing chemicals:

Play smart. Wear long sleeves and pants, and stay indoors at dusk, when mosquitoes come out.

Use natural repellents. Despite the ubiquity of citronella and herbal products, a test published in the *New England Journal of Medicine* demonstrated that they kept mosquitoes away for less than twenty minutes. The only natural product whose effectiveness exceeded one hour is a soybean oil product called Bite Blocker for Kids, which the U.S. Department of Agriculture found to be as effective as a 15 percent concentration of DEET and lasted for four to eight hours. The botanical product Repel, with lemon eucalyptus derivatives, was found by the CDC to be as effective as low concentrations of DEET.

Make your garden repellent. Near your home, plant scented geraniums, lemon thyme, marigold, citrosa plants, sweet basil, and/or sassafras. In ponds or other water features (that don't contain fish), use mosquito dunks or disks containing *Bacillus thuringiensis israelensis* (found in garden stores), bacteria that kill mosquito larvae.

Spare the DEET. If you go the DEET route—and you may need to, if West Nile virus or equine encephalitis virus is detected in your area— then choose the lowest concentration, less than 10 percent, which should provide up to two hours of protection. Be sure always to read the DEET label. Apply sparingly or spray on clothes (for example, the cuffs and neck of the shirt) instead of skin. Never spray a child's face and keep it off hands. Shower when you get home, or change clothes and wash skin with a soapy cloth when you've crawled into the tent for the night.

🌀 Expert Opinion 🌀
Raspberries Changed My Life
By Myra Goodman, cofounder of Earthbound Farm, author of
Food to Live By: The Earthbound Farm Organic Cookbook

When I was growing up in New York City, fed on TV dinners and sugary cereal, I never gave a thought to how food was produced. In my neighborhood, there was one teeny health-food store that carried pockmarked, shriveled apples and a couple of limp carrots.

Then I went to California for college, as did my husband (we met in high school), and we took a year off before grad school. To earn tuition money, we stumbled on an opportunity to live on a little raspberry farm and do repairs in exchange for rent. We had no farming experience. The guy who lived there previously gave us a crash course in how to care for raspberries. He showed us the chemical shed and pointed out the dormant spray and fertilizer and how to put it into the drip line. But when it came time to start applying the chemicals, we had a very instinctive reaction. This was a time when most people didn't know what "organic" meant, but when you're the person who's going to handle chemicals, breathe them, apply them to your farm, then eat food grown with them and sell it to people who come to your farm stand, you realize, "These chemicals actually kill pests and weeds." That was our wake-up call.

At the local nursery we got Rodale's *Encyclopedia of Organic Gardening*, and got hooked into the world of what many people considered "hippie farming." Eventually we moved on from raspberries and came up with something else we thought we could grow efficiently on a small farm: baby lettuces. That was our first big success, and the turning point in our company.

Since we started back in 1984, so much information on the problems of conventionally produced food has shown that our intuition was right. Though organic is more expensive to farm, it's a better value when you account for the effect on the environment and on health.

Later, when we were farming more land and had our children, we started to garden at home again. I have the cutest video of my little boy when he was two and my daughter was five, with their shovels and gloves, where you can hear my son with his lispy voice talking about all the different things that we were planting that year.

Now my kids are teenagers and they're both smart eaters. They understand better than most of their peers how their food is grown, what's in season and why it tastes better, how the changing weather affects the farm. I believe you should make educating your kids about food a priority, like teaching them good hygiene and street safety. I see the awakening all the time in school groups that come through. Kids on our tours will pick some fresh English peas, open them and eat them, and all of a sudden peas are their favorite vegetable. Same thing with a really ripe cantaloupe or apple.

The nature in your own little backyard garden is full of miracles. There's the miracle of planting a seed and watering it and watching it grow, and then there's the sadness when it gets eaten by snails or a gopher. For kids, it's so fun and healthy to go outside and weed versus sitting in front of the TV. Or to see if the string beans are ready and pick them for dinner (even if your string beans are growing in a pot on your fire escape). Gardening gets kids in touch with nature, gets them using their bodies, gets them excited about trying new things and eating healthy fresh food. In a supermarket, you see very few varieties of produce: a few different apples, one type of carrot. When you garden you can get a seed catalog and see how there aren't just orange carrots, but yellow carrots and white ones. Look at how many kinds of tomatoes there are, how some have to be trellised and some are bushes.

For kids the most exciting thing is pulling things out of the earth. Radishes are the quickest gratification; carrots take a little longer, but everyone falls in love with them. Potatoes are the most exciting of all! Harvesting potatoes is like an Easter egg hunt. You loosen the soil so they can dig their hands around and find all shapes and sizes like buried treasure. If kids' first experiences with food are so amazing, they're going to love to eat fresh produce. So there's no more powerful way to introduce the idea than by growing it in or around your house. You realize how long it takes to pick a pound of string beans and to grow it, and all the challenges of keeping it watered and fertilized and pest-free. You have more of an appreciation of your food—and your planet.

Step # 6. Start a Kids' Garden

Perhaps the best way to stimulate kids to live a more ecologically aware life is to help them grow a green thumb. The world becomes a great science experiment, and there's a huge sense of accomplishment from growing, picking, and eating your own food. Kim Graham-Nye, cofounder of gDiapers, tells of how, while visiting her mother in the Canadian countryside, she and her four-year-old son, Flynn, went to the garden before dinner—where he proceeded to do something he'd never done before.

"He ate peas," she recounts. "Fresh green peas and lots of them. Of course, we'd offered him green peas thousands of times before, but this was different. It was the first time he'd stood in a garden and picked them himself."

When kids realize that their food comes from the ground, not from the fridge or grocery store, it changes them. They sense that Mother Nature may actually *need* them. And, as Graham-Nye says, "gardening means playing in the dirt, so intangible and lofty lessons aside, kids just love it!" She offers her checklist for getting kids interested in growing, and eating, their own veggies:

- **Let the sunshine in.** Make sure your garden gets plenty of sun.
- **Grow anywhere.** If you can't go right into the ground, use a kiddie pool, sandbox, or large pots on a deck. Make sure your container has holes for drainage.
- **Start planting.** April or May, after the threat of frost, is recommended for most plant hardiness zones.
- **Stake a sign.** Make a sign for each family member and stake it into the ground or pot, dividing the garden so everyone gets a section.
- **Select fast-growing vegetables.** Tomatoes, snow peas, cucumbers, beans, peppers, and carrots work well, but ultimately let the children choose what to plant in their own garden. If there's room, grow pumpkins—they'll be ready for Halloween.
- **Add some bright flowers.** Cosmos, sunflowers, and zinnia are popular annuals that will bloom throughout the growing season.
- **Do some of the prep yourself.** If your children are young, prepare the soil, then bring the kids in for the digging and planting.
- **Make a ritual of watering.** Do a bug count, check for earthworms, chart a plant's growth. Keep kids engaged in the cultivation process.
- **Bring it together.** At dinnertime, send them to the garden to select the veggies.

Step #7. Check Your Deck and Play Set

Backyard decks have proliferated wildly over the last couple of decades as grill-happy homeowners erect outdoor living rooms. But most of these wooden structures—as well as picnic tables, treehouses, and play sets—contain an unwelcome dinner guest: arsenic. The arsenic in pressure-treated wood is part of a formula—which also includes chromium and copper—called CCA, which was designed to kill wood-chewing insects and fungi that cause rot. Although arsenic was used for centuries as a poison, the main concern about it today is the potential cancer risk to kids who are exposed. The Environmental Working Group has shown that high levels of arsenic leach out of pressure-treated wood for years after installation—which happens when rain pools on it, bringing arsenic to the surface. The EWG also found that the amount of arsenic that testers wiped off an area of wood—about the size of a four-year-old's hand—exceeded what the EPA allows in a glass of water. Just as worrisome, arsenic in the soil from 40 percent of backyards or parks tested exceeds EPA's Superfund cleanup levels. (Superfund sites are the nastiest, most toxic, polluted areas across the nation—our parks and backyards should not resemble them.) If your deck or other backyard structure was built before 2005, there's a good chance it contains CCA. Go to safe2play.org or call 510-594-9864 to order a twenty-dollar home test kit to measure potential exposure from a CCA wood surface; or order a kit from the EWG (ewg.org/reports/poisonwoodrivals/orderform.php). You can also chip a piece off your deck and send it to a state-certified environmental testing lab.

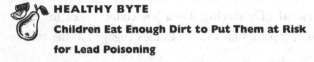

HEALTHY BYTE
Children Eat Enough Dirt to Put Them at Risk for Lead Poisoning

The main way children get lead into their bodies is by ingesting contaminated soil or house dust. In fact, children under the age of six eat a relatively large amount of dirt. Some toddlers will actually stick an occasional handful into their mouth. Even if they spit it out, a lot of lead gets left behind and swallowed. Now, you may be saying, "My child doesn't eat dirt, so I don't have to worry." The fact is, even normal activity brings dirty little fingers or play objects into the mouth. In risk assessment, we assume young children ingest 200 milligrams of soil a day, about the amount of soil in a fine coating on a teaspoon. Not a lot, yet enough to introduce toxic amounts into children if their yard is contaminated by lead or other toxins such as arsenic. Bottom line, if you have an older house (pre-1978) and young children, you need to be especially vigilant for lead paint, inside and out.

Source: What's Toxic, What's Not *by Dr. Gary Ginsberg and Brian Toal, M.S.P.H.*

Seal your deal. If you find that your deck is CCA-treated and you're not in a position to rebuild, the Safe Playgrounds Project recommends that you seal it with two coats of semitransparent oil-based deck stain and reseal at least once a year.

Scrub up. Make sure children wash their hands well after touching CCA-treated lumber and never eat while on an unsealed CCA deck.

Build a better deck. Some woods, like cedar and redwood, are naturally rot-resistant. If these are too costly, then opt for recycled-content composite decking materials, which are made from recycled plastic and wood pulp and often look a lot like real wood. Any home improvement store can talk you through the options. Also, avoid railroad ties, which contain creosote—basically toxic tar.

Avoid utility poles. Wood utility poles are treated with harmful chemicals, including CCA and creosote. Salvage companies sometimes give away older poles for garden and residential use—steer clear.

Check your outdoor furniture. Some older deck and garden furniture may also have been made from pressure-treated wood or other chemically laced compositions. If you're not sure what kind of wood you've got, you can refinish it once a year with a water-based sealant to keep any contaminants inside. If you're buying new, some nontoxic and eco-friendly materials for outdoor furniture include recycled wood, environmentally farmed teak, composite plastics, or, if you're looking for something as-is, recycled plastic furniture. If using painted cast-iron furniture that's more than a couple decades old, there's a chance you've got lead paint on your patio. You can perform a basic lead test with a kit bought at a hardware store. (It provides a basic reading but may not be the most accurate.) If you've got little ones, consider different furniture.

Find safe sand. Some play sand used in sandboxes and around swing sets contains tremolite (a form of asbestos) or very fine crystalline silica; the most dangerous of these is made from crushed quarry rock. The kind of sand you *want* in your box—the safest and most natural—is washed beach or river sand that is fairly granular, not powder-fine. For years, manufacturers of toy sand have successfully lobbied the Consumer Product Safety Commission to keep labeling to indicate its source off of sand, so it's difficult to gauge safety by looking at the bag. Don't buy sand unless the manufacturer can assure you that it consists of beach or river sand, and that it's not quarry rock. See Healthy Resources for brands.

Step #8. Use Safe Playgrounds

Sandra Steingraber, renowned biologist and writer, discovered that her daughter's nursery school wooden playground equipment tested positive for arsenic at levels far greater than the state-mandated clean-up standard. The school's plan to seal the play structure and replace the mulch under and around it didn't satisfy Dr. Steingraber, a cancer survivor, so she enrolled her daughter in a different school. "Poisoning our children and poisoning the land should not be a consequence of childhood play," she wrote of her decision in the *Ithaca Journal*.

Another potential health risk in playgrounds is lead. In a study on the safety of thousands of playgrounds, the U.S. Public Interest Research Group and Consumer Federation of America found that half of the playgrounds they tested had peeling, chipping, or cracking paint on equipment surfaces. Kids run the risk of ingesting lead if they put their hands in their mouths after touching peeling paint or paint chips.

Most playgrounds in public parks and spaces are now being built from safer materials such as steel or recycled plastic (sometimes made from old milk jugs). Avoid letting your kids play on older equipment with chipped or peeling paint. If you're concerned about whether your neighborhood playground is contaminated, visit safe2play.org for information about community action.

Parentblog

Field of Dreams?

By Tanya Murphy, environmental health activist

In the last several years, hundreds of synthetic-turf athletic fields have been installed around the country for our children to play on. You've probably seen them—roughly a three-inch-thick carpet of ground-up recycled tires over AstroTurf.

I'd read online about how two professors had taken samples from one such field in New York City and identified worrisome levels of irritants, heavy metals, and known carcinogens. One day, while driving through the Connecticut town next to ours, I noticed one of these types of fields. I got out of my car, walked toward the field and right away noticed the smell of tires. I knelt down, scooped up a handful of little granules, and they left a stain on my hands. *Kids are playing on this?* I thought. I couldn't help but ask: How might something like ground-up tires affect human beings, especially children?

I contacted a group called Environment and Human Health, Inc. (EHHI), which had detailed the health risks associated with pesticides; EHHI worked with Connecticut state legislators to get pesticides banned from playing fields and schools. EHHI conducted its own test of samples taken from a local playing field, and their findings were similar to the professors': They identified four heavy metals and several known carcinogens. Studies of rubber-granule fields in numerous countries have raised red flags about health risks potentially caused by these fields. (One oft-cited study that concludes that the rubber granules are safe was conducted by the French government body charged with figuring out how to recycle used tires.)

I don't know what the risks are or aren't. But environmental dangers play no favorites. I feel incredibly grateful for the health of my children, but isn't health every child's birthright?

Step #9. Swimming in It: Maintaining a Deep Green Pool

Chlorine in swimming pools kills bacteria and other microorganisms in water but can be inhaled or absorbed and cause irritated skin and burning eyes. It can also lead to respiratory problems and an increased risk of asthma. The less of it you use, the better. Don't drop chlorine tablets into the water (they can produce high concentrations of chlorine that increase health risks). Test your water frequently to avoid overchlorinating and maintain the proper level.

Several new, less toxic methods have been developed for reducing or eliminating chlorine. These can all be quite expensive and may not suit every system, so before you switch, consult with your pool maintenance company.

- **Salt.** A salt generator produces its own chlorine (high school chem reminder: salt = sodium + chlorine) so that you don't have to keep putting in more. The volume of salt added to the pool is relatively minor so, no, your pool won't become sea-salty.
- **Ultraviolet light.** UV light disinfects; some chemical treatment is still required but chlorine can be reduced by up to 70 percent.

- **Ozonators.** A form of oxygen that kills bacteria and viruses faster than chlorine. An ozone system won't completely eliminate the need for chlorine but reduces it by roughly 80 percent.

Note: Both ozone and UV are very dangerous to humans; they kill tiny bacteria but people should have no direct exposure themselves.

For conservation purposes, a safety cover reduces evaporation by up to 90 percent. You might also look into energy-saving filtration pumps and solar water heaters.

Step #10. Leave the Outdoors Out

Eighty-five percent of the dirt in homes is brought in from the outside, on our shoe bottoms or the paws of pets. The EPA's "Doormat Study" has shown that virtually all lead dust inside homes is caused by lead-contaminated soil from outside. Of all the tips in this book, perhaps none will be simpler than this: Remove your shoes when you come in. You protect your floors, especially carpeting, from the mostly invisible enemies on your shoe bottoms—dirt, chemicals, bacteria, feces, lead dust, pesticides, allergenic dust, animal dander, and other pollutants.

If you can keep your shoes from crossing the threshold, great; if not, get a straw mat. Wiping shoes on a mat and removing them at the door cuts lead dust by 60 percent. Keep some slippers by the entrance for you and houseguests, to ensure that what happens outside stays outside.

And everyone should wash hands when they come in. The physical act of washing with soap and water removes all kinds of microorganisms, including the viruses that cause colds and flu.

 ONE STEP BEYOND

Get Rid of Your Lawn. Join the millions of people who are giving up the battle against their lawn and planting instead with native perennial ground covers and grasses. Investigate the "Smaller American Lawns Today" (SALT) movement—started by Dr. William Niering, a botany professor at Connecticut College—by clicking on arboretum.conncoll.edu/salt/salt.html for more information.

Build a Worm Farm with Your Kids. By creating your own worm compost bin, you turn your kitchen garbage into nutrient-rich food for your plants. Your kids will love helping, mostly because worms are involved. To set up a worm compost bin at home, you need only an opaque container with a lid (a 10-gallon plastic one will do); a drill to make air holes; shredded newspaper; and dirt, water, and worms which, if you don't have them in your yard, can be bought at bait shops (red wigglers—*Eisenia fetida*—are best) or ordered online. For all you need to know about making a worm compost bin, see the Earthbound Farm site, ebfarm.com, and search "worm composting."

CHAPTER 7

Every Sip—and Breath—You Take

CLEAN WATER AND AIR SOLUTIONS

I t's elemental, and elementary: Almost nothing in our physical world warrants our care more than the water we drink and the air we breathe. As ever, kids are far more affected by both, good and bad. In the first six months of life, pound for pound, a child drinks seven times more liquid than an adult; the air intake of a resting infant is double that of a grown-up. And with each sip and breath children take, their bodies are more vulnerable to unwanted chemicals in these elements.

Who among us, even the most tree-hugging optimists, doesn't sometimes feel helpless about how to keep our planet's air and water clean—with coal-burning power plants being built in abundance in certain developing (and developed) countries, with everything from toxic waste and spilled oil to flushed chemicals tainting our waterways? I know I do. However, you absolutely can make significant, immediate improvements to your water and air *indoors,* where we spend 90 percent of our time, and where the concentration of pollutants in the air is two to five times greater, on average, than outdoors—and where the water is sometimes not as pure as we would hope.

But ensuring clean water and air is not as straightforward as, say, identifying unwanted ingredients in food. Yes, there are lots of tests available to measure the purity of these elements, but not enough to cover the thousands of chemicals registered for use. There's an abundance of choices of water and air filters on the market, but you'll want first to understand your own home's particular roster of contaminants and issues before taking steps. Still, while each of us must identify our own solutions, some solutions work for everyone.

PART ONE: WATER, WATER EVERYWHERE

Step #1. Run Cold

When you first turn on the water in the morning, run the cold tap for about a minute to help flush pipes. Lead can leach into water that sits overnight in plumbing, particularly in older houses. Lead is particularly toxic to kids and has been linked to decreased intelligence and developmental disabilities. If opening the spigot offends your conservationist's sensibility, buy an inexpensive water filter (see Step #3) and forget this tip.

Since many contaminants are more apt to leach into hot tap water than cold, use cold water for cooking, drinking, or—very important— mixing infant formula. Hot water heaters/boilers tend to accumulate sediment and contamination, and the high temperature provides the perfect brew for biological and chemical pollutants to flourish.

HEALTHY BYTE
Boiling Water Is No Cure-All

Boiling water zaps bacteria, which is why we sterilize with it. But those who reuse kettle water to conserve are better off starting with a fresh supply from the cold faucet because evaporation may slightly increase lead concentration. And pediatricians agree that anyone with a normal public water source has no need to boil water to prepare infant formula.

Step #2. Test Your Water

Water helps us maintain our internal ecosystem by replenishing cells, encouraging brain health and activity, and basically every other human function. Fortunately, the U.S. water supply is among the safest in the world. Some pollutants and sediment—picked up by water as it courses through bedrock and soil, sopping up industrial and agricultural runoff— are filtered out by municipal treatment plants. Then chemicals such as chlorine are added to kill the kind of bacteria that used to cause water-borne epidemics like typhoid. However, in some homes and municipalities the water may not be as pure as we would hope. And the bad news about chlorine is that it reacts with organic materials already present in water to form traces of chemical by-products called THMs (trihalomethanes), which are carcinogens.

To address drinking water safety, the EPA has set maximum contaminant levels (MCLs) for public drinking water (not private wells). Your local public supplier has to provide you with an annual drinking water quality report (known also as a Consumer Confidence Report) that usually arrives with your bill and lists the chemicals and parasites they test for, their levels, federal limits, and how the water is treated.

For peace of mind, you might consider having your water tested anyway because concentrations of some elements—lead, for example—may vary significantly from home to home. Testing your water is relatively simple, quick, and cheap.

Do it yourself. Basic, trustworthy water-testing devices such as the WaterSafe kit are available online or at hardware stores, starting at under twenty dollars, and allow you to test quickly for bacteria, lead, some pesticides, chlorine, pH, and hardness. Results for most contaminants are available in ten minutes or less, while bacteria results take two days. (For more information on test options, see oasisdesign.net and watercenter.com.) If any of your levels exceed government standards, call the EPA's Safe Drinking Water Hotline at 800-426-4791.

Or call in the pros. If you want total reassurance, then by all means let a professional lab test your water, though it can cost upward of $150. For a list of state-certified labs, visit epa.gov/safewater/labs/index.html.

Test your well water. The EPA recommends you test well water annually, particularly for nitrate and coliform bacteria (yes, poop, from animals or leaky septic tanks). Take precautions not to do anything to contaminate your well, like dump motor oil, paint, varnish, fertilizers, or pesticides on your property. Be aware of groundwater pollution sources in your neighborhood, like a nearby gas station, chemical plant, or farm. (If you live on a farm or near one, test your water twice a year to watch for pesticide level spikes during heavier application times.) Again, you can do the test yourself or have a state-certified lab or other qualified expert do it. If you discover contaminants above recommended levels, call your local health agency and/or talk to your doctor to find out next steps.

260
number of contaminants detected in water, over half of which have no safety standards.
(Environmental Working Group, 2005)

If you rely on a neighborhood or community well, try to get neighbors to agree not to use pesticides, fertilizers, and other chemicals near the supply source—generally within one-half mile (though pesticides have migrated farther both in surface and groundwater).

Step #3. Find a Filter

Once your water is tested, you'll have a better idea of what you're dealing with. Today's filters remove the vast majority of unwanted impurities from tap water. If your results exceed the federal standard for a particular contaminant, filter for it. If your results are okay but you want reassurance, filter anyway—it can't hurt. First, though, it may help to speak with a toxicologist or the EPA's Safe Drinking Water Hotline

(800-426-4791) to understand the issues. There are many types of filters from which to choose.

Carbon filter (pitcher or container). If you put your water only through a carbon adsorption, Brita-type pitcher filter (whose activated carbon, by the way, comes from coconut shells), you'll knock out most of the chlorine, coarse sediment, and organic chemicals. It's an easy, inexpensive fix (as little as twenty dollars) that, alone, vastly improves your water quality. It will not, however, remove pesticides, microbes, and most heavy metals.

Faucet-mounted filter. These units attach right to a faucet or head and typically also use the carbon adsorption method. They work great on bathroom sinks, since they're small and can't handle the demands of the kitchen.

Kitchen countertop unit. This diverts water away from the regular tap via a hose to the filter unit, where some contaminants get trapped. These units typically use reverse osmosis to filter water, which can handle higher volumes and work like hot water heaters where a reservoir of filtered water is stored in a tank. The filter removes more contaminants than a carbon system but can be expensive ($300 to $3,000) and, unless you're really handy, needs to be professionally installed.

Whole-house filter. For purists or those whose water supply comes from a well or spring, this is the most heavy-duty system out there and is installed where water enters the house plumbing. *All* the water in your house will be filtered—not just the water from one or two taps—and you'll need to change only one filter. However, these are expensive (at least $1,500) and require company installation.

Distiller. This fairly low-tech system softens water by removing minerals as well as heavy metals, nitrates, bacteria, and viruses. It won't remove pesticides, THMs, or chlorine, and it requires dedication on your part: You have to boil the water, plus there's more cleaning required. These tend to be much cheaper, though—roughly $250.

For recommended brands and more information, see Healthy Resources. No matter which system you choose, maintain it. If you don't, you run the risk of bacteria or sediment buildup, which sort of defeats the point.

Step #4. Bottle Your Own

Forget, for a moment, that the booming bottled water business is a huge environmental nightmare: that 137 million petroleum-based plastic bottles pile up in landfills every day and take at least one thousand years to decompose, not to mention the somewhat ludicrous fact that rivers of truck fuel are being burned to transport drinking water to areas with perfectly fine drinking water (some is even flown in from Fiji!). From a health standpoint alone, when you drink bottled water you're often feeding your body a resource that's available at higher quality—and free—right from your own tap. In a four-year study, the Natural Resources Defense Council found that the water from one-third of the 103 bottled waters tested were actually of *lower* quality than public tap water. Bottled water is required to be tested less frequently than tap water for bacteria and chemical contaminants, and doesn't have to adhere to the same standards for content.

One more thing: Ever wonder why bottled water has an expiration date? It's not because the water goes bad but because the plastic degrades over time, releasing chemicals into the water. Hardened polycarbonate plastic #7 is often the choice for five-gallon jugs and some smaller water bottles (as well as clear plastic baby bottles). Polycarbonate can leach its primary building block—the suspected hormone disruptor Bisphenol A—into the liquid; the hotter or older it gets, the likelier the leaching. If you leave a water bottle in the car, baking in the sun, don't drink from it later. And don't refill plastic bottles, since the plastic can wear down from multiple uses.

Safer plastic designations to look for on water bottles: #1, #2, #4, and #5. (Make it a mantra: *1-2-4-5, 1-2-4-5 . . .*) All things being equal, #1 is best because it's more easily recycled or remanufactured than others, releases fewer emissions during manufacture, and leaves less solid waste.

Of course, it's the portability of bottled water that we all appreciate. Every morning before work, I fill my two forty-ounce, stainless steel Klean Kanteens with filtered water from the home tap. Look up other reusable metal water bottles in the Healthy Resources section.

Step #5. Waste Not

Because water seems so plentiful, we tend to use more than we truly need—a great deal more. But appearances are misleading. If one gallon of water represents all the water on the planet, a half cup of that would represent freshwater, and a mere one drop of that is what's available to us (the rest is frozen in ice caps or locked in aquifers deep underground). According to the U.S. Geological Survey, less than 0.3 percent of the world's water is usable for drinking, washing, bathing, and other human purposes, so we should be conserving more than we do. I love washing my car by hand, hardly the most efficient use of this precious resource, and I admit to indulging occasionally in a long hot shower. But whatever our individual H_2O weaknesses, there are ways to offset overconsumption.

You already know the classic, finger-wagging admonitions: *Don't let faucets run as you brush your teeth. . . . Water lawns sparingly. . . . Shower rather than bathe. . . . If it's yellow, let it mellow. . . .* Here are some lesser-known but effective steps to reduce water use:

Install faucet aerators and low-flow showerheads and toilets. Reducing flow in sinks, showers, and toilets is, when taken together, arguably the single most effective way to conserve water. A low-flow, one-and-a-half-gallon-per-minute head allows you to indulge in a five-minute bit of heaven because it uses less than half the water of a conventional, four- to five-gallon-per-minute head. And if you replace the regular eighteen-liter-per-flush toilet with an ultralow volume one—about six liters per flush—you save over 20 percent of your *total* indoor water use. You can self-install aerators (for around ten dollars) and low-flow showerheads (around thirty to fifty dollars); low-flow toilets cost about five hundred dollars, installed. You can also get a hands-free faucet (pedalvalve.com), which reduces consumption by allowing you to turn off the water even when your hands are occupied.

4:1
approximate ratio
of water used for a
typical bath to that
used for a five-
minute shower
(using a conven-
tional shower
head).
(Environmental
Protection Agency,
2007)

Water your garden and yard in the early morning or night. Because there's less evaporation then, more water goes into the ground.

Set the dishwasher for "energy-saving" or "light wash." These conservation modes use less water and run for less time. If dishes are really soiled, of course, then go for the more powerful setting; you don't want to have to run the load a second time.

Keep a cold one going. If you prefer your drinking water icy-cold, keep a pitcher of it in the fridge. It saves on all that tap water we waste each time we stand there, thirsty, waiting for the stream to chill.

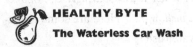 **HEALTHY BYTE**
The Waterless Car Wash

Started by a mom with a chemically sensitive child, Green Earth Waterless Car Wash (greenearthcarwash.com) sells an effective, simple-to-use product that can save hundreds of gallons per use; it's biodegradable; dye-, VOC-, and fragrance-free; and made with organic coconut soaps.

In addition to conserving a supremely limited and vital natural resource, using less water in your home means releasing fewer contaminants into your air. (Pollutants in water escape into the air from the dishwasher, toilet, and shower.) Which leads us back to the issue of breathing easier.

PART TWO: CLEARING THE AIR

One supposed achievement of modern living is an airtight home, outfitted with powerful air-conditioning and an energy-efficient central heating system that keep noise, dirt, and foul weather safely outside its double-glazed panes. Hermetically sealing ourselves in our houses may reduce fuel consumption, but it also traps and recirculates air pollution—particles, allergens, and harmful chemicals. It's almost like some bad horror movie in which the hero bolts the door against some invading alien only to discover *it's already in the house!*

Since we spend most of our time indoors, it's no surprise that the EPA has named indoor air quality one of the top five environmental risks to public health. When we were young, most of us could count on one hand the kids we knew who suffered from asthma. Now we can't keep track. Since 1985, rates of childhood asthma have more than doubled, and continue to grow.

Even if you keep a pretty clean home, air pollutants are circulated by many sources discussed in other chapters: chemicals in cleaning products, synthetic fragrances, paint, carpets, and furniture; tiny, easily inhaled particles resulting from mold, bacteria, mites, pollen, and other biological pollutants; and irritants released in smoke from stoves, cigarettes, fireplaces, and candles. While outdoor air pollution is beyond our immediate control, there are many easy changes to make to clean the air inside your home so your family can collectively take a deep breath.

Parentblog
On Having a Child with Asthma
By Michelle Obama, hospital executive, wife of
Illinois Senator Barack Obama

One afternoon about six years ago we were at the circus with our daughter Malia, who was then three. We noticed she was having trouble breathing. As the circus went on, Malia's ability to breathe got worse, so we took her to the emergency room. It was scary. She's our first child, and we were learning a lot about parenting on the job. And you never want to see your child sick or struggling.

That was the day we found out she had asthma. Since then, we've worked to stay ahead of it, so she's more comfortable. We take Malia to the pediatrician regularly to ensure she has whatever treatment she requires. She had an inhaler for a while, but hasn't needed one for a year or two now. We keep our house dust- and dander-free, and don't bring anything in that will disrupt her. One of the deals we made as a family when we decided to enter the Presidential race was that the girls could get a dog. Malia researched all kinds of dogs that are hypoallergenic, so the dog doesn't upset her breathing.

Our family is lucky to have access to quality health care and the resources to cover the costs, so that Malia's asthma can be treated and so that she can be a kid—staying focused on her passions, like soccer and reading, and not letting asthma get in her way.

But asthma is not so easily dealt with by all parents. Many parents don't know the causes or how to treat the symptoms. Others can't afford either preventive care or treatment. For many more, they can't get away from their jobs or simply have too much else to worry about in their daily lives that they can't get their children to the doctor. So time goes by, the issue gets worse, and they end up crowding emergency rooms for ailments that are then out of control. By then the condition may be more life-threatening, requiring treatment that's more intense—and expensive.

Parents of children with asthma need to know how to reduce the chances of an attack, how to treat an attack if it happens, and when to go to the hospital. Irritants and allergens in the air, such as smoke, dust mites, pet dander, cockroaches, mold, and pollen, can make attacks more likely. So parents who have children with asthma should keep houses clean of potential triggers.

But that's not all of it. The number of children with asthma has more than doubled since the 1980s, and this epidemic disproportionately affects minority communities. As a society, we need to help parents in the inner city live in clean environments that aren't dangerous to their children's health. There are both genetic and environmental factors to asthma, but genetics change too slowly to explain the spike in cases we've seen recently. Clearly we're not doing a good enough job addressing the environmental causes. Air pollution triggers symptoms. The state of some of our inner-city housing is clearly unhealthy.

From my experience in health care, I know that a lot of what contributes to the crisis is people not taking adequate care of themselves on the front end. In addition to living in unhealthy communities, our children eat poorly and exercise less than they should. They spend more time indoors, in front of the TV, where so many other asthma triggers reside. All of this together weakens their immune systems. So we need to make our children's environments healthier. Nearly one-third of Americans live in neighborhoods without sidewalks and less than half of our country's children have a playground within walking distance of their homes.

In the long term, community-based prevention efforts, which have helped to drive down rates of smoking and lead poisoning—to give two encouraging examples—are underused despite their effectiveness. Less than four cents of every health-care dollar is spent on prevention and public health. Our health-care system has become a disease-care system, and the time for change is well overdue.

Malia's nine years old now. Just recently she brought up the circus and her asthma attack to us. She seems to remember the whole thing pretty clearly, which is incredible. She was three then, and it made quite an impression on her.

Step #6. Beat Allergy and Asthma at the Source

Allergies can be pinned to a variety of factors, including genetics and environmental exposures resulting in hypersensitivity to allergens. The immune system is behind all this: Its job is to act like a nightclub bouncer for foreign intruders, such as bacteria and viruses, identifying them and keeping them out. In the case of allergies, however, our systems may overreact to something fairly benign, such as pollen, which doesn't provide a direct threat the way, say, a virus can. All that wheezing, sneezing, and eye watering is the body's attempt to rid itself of the intruder, which can be exhausting for allergy sufferers, not to mention extremely disruptive (according to the American Academy of Allergy, Asthma and Immunology, allergic rhinitis or hay fever accounts for 2 million lost days of school annually).

6.5 million number of American children affected by asthma. (Centers for Disease Control and Prevention, 2005)

For some, though, allergic reactions can be quite severe, from acute asthma attacks to anaphylactic shock. While genetics may assume some of the responsibility for the recent spike in asthma, environmental exposure increasingly looks like a major culprit.

Hundreds of different allergens float around in our air. One type we can effectively control in our home environments is "biological"—that is, triggers that result from the big and small creatures with whom we coexist. These triggers, such as mold, bacteria, dander, and cockroach waste, thrive on food and moisture. How to minimize your family's exposure?

Detonate dust mites. They're microscopic, their droppings even smaller. Yet that's enough to make them potent allergens for some children and, according to a National Academy of Sciences report, to trigger the development of asthma in susceptible children. The mites live by eating dead skin cells that flake off of bodies, and so they tend to thrive in bedrooms and living rooms. They also love moisture. A few ways to limit mites: Encase mattresses and pillows with impermeable covers; avoid feather comforters and pillows where mites love to wallow; wash bedding in very hot water (130°F); and dry sheets and blankets in a hot dryer for an extra few minutes. If you can give up some carpets and curtains, that's great since kids get into them, roll on them, and press their faces into them. If you can't, then vacuum frequently, using a machine with a HEPA filter.

Run a clean, tight (lidded) ship. Starve roaches, whose body parts and waste are common allergy triggers, by cleaning up all crumbs and food residue and by sweeping the kitchen after meals, wiping down counters, and sealing foods tightly. Don't leave water standing in the sink and make sure you have a tightly lidded garbage can. Mounds of dirty clothes are a haven for mites and mildew, while stacks of newspaper provide a welcome mat for cockroaches. (For healthy pest control ideas, see Chapter 2.)

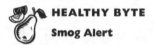

HEALTHY BYTE
Smog Alert

How unfair is this? Smog is usually worst between 3 and 6 P.M.—in other words, exactly when kids are apt to be playing outdoors. Doctors advise that asthmatic children refrain from exertion outside when it's hot and smoggy or a dusty wind is blowing. Visit airnow.gov to find out about air quality conditions and sign up for e-mail alerts.

Dry out. If humidity drops below 50 percent, mold and dust mites can't grow. Dehumidifiers and air conditioners help in areas that are consistently damp. Try to keep humidity levels between 30 and 50 percent, which you can measure with a store-bought hygrometer (it costs twenty to thirty dollars). Repair leaky plumbing, seal cracks in basement floors and walls, and ventilate when showering and cooking.

Minimize pet dander. Animal dander is just dead skin flakes or cat saliva that evaporates and then invades our space. Short of getting rid of your pet (not that I'm suggesting that, though in some cases it *is* necessary), wash him frequently without letting his skin dry out, perhaps with an eco-safe conditioner. Improving your pet's diet can also help (see Chapter 8 for more information on keeping your pet's skin well-conditioned). And by all means keep Snowbell out of the bedroom; buy mattress and pillow encasements to keep dander from penetrating; change or wash the animal's bed or favorite spots; opt for bare floors or area rugs over carpet; and cover bedroom vents with dense filtering material like cheesecloth, so that air-conditioning and forced-air heating doesn't spread animal allergens all over the house. If your rugs cannot be machine-washed, then throw them into the dryer with no heat to remove built-up dust and dander on a regular basis.

Replace filters. Furnace and heating-duct filters collect dust and mold and should be changed regularly (the frequency depends on type and model).

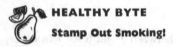

HEALTHY BYTE
Stamp Out Smoking!

There are four thousand or more chemicals in cigarette smoke, and research shows that secondhand smoke increases a child's risk of developing ear and respiratory infections, asthma, cancer, and sudden infant death syndrome. Kick smokers outside; if a neighbor's smoke is wafting into your house, ask him (nicely) to smoke elsewhere in his home.

Open wide. Once again, many homes built in the last twenty or more years are amazingly well-sealed, trapping air pollutants and moisture indoors. Add to this the many chemical vapors that get stuck inside and pose respiratory risks—perfumes, air fresheners, carpet, etc. So open windows for at least five minutes a day—the more, the better—even if only a crack in the winter, to circulate air and let indoor pollutants out. On hot, humid days, however, shut windows and ventilate instead with air conditioners. (The benefit to individual health surely outweighs the environmental detriment.)

Parentblog
The Double-Edged Sword
By Brooke Shields, actress

When you make choices to live better, greener, and more organic, it's not always so clear-cut; that is, you want to do the right thing but you also have to do what works for you and your lifestyle. Sometimes that means choosing the lesser of two evils. An example from when I was a teenager: In 1982, I got a job at the San Diego Zoo working with wild cats. Every day we fed them so much meat that eventually something in me just snapped and I didn't want to eat meat anymore. For thirteen years, I was a vegetarian—no beef, no fowl. I was doing a good thing, I thought, a virtuous thing. But over time, I felt weaker and weaker. I wasn't getting enough protein, my doctor told me. In 1995 I was in Russia and I saw these chicken kebabs…and I took a bite. Suddenly I felt like I was a balloon in the Macy's Thanksgiving Day parade, being lifted up by animal protein. I so desperately needed that protein. Other people don't. The morning I got pregnant I woke up screaming for beef. At least I try to make it organic.

When you become a parent, you would think the choices become more obvious, and they do—you always know who comes first—but then there are still trade-offs; there always are. I switched to chlorine-free diapers for my daughter. They're better for the environment but not as absorbent as the Elmo diapers she was wearing. Do I live greener and use the chlorine-free diapers all the time, including at night, when she pees more, and I lose sleep because I have to change her in the middle of the night because they can't hold as much? Or do I use the Elmo diapers just for the nighttime, sleep through the night, and put her in the environmentally friendly kind during the day? You do all you can but there are particulars to your own life that you must respect. I've changed all our products to eco-friendly ones but sometimes I have to bring in something less eco-friendly as a supplement. I use all recycled paper products except toilet paper. It's like: You want the hybrid but then you're driving your kids around in this gas-guzzling tank of a car that makes you feel safe…which is ironic, of course, because it's cars like that that contribute more to something that doesn't make us feel safe for our children.

I've gone in both directions. First, it's, *Okay I'm going to do this completely.* Then something happens, I feel guilty about how much electricity and water my home uses and I think, *What's the point?* It's a real psychological battle. Plus, I'm the type where, if someone from an organization— Save the This or Save the That—makes me feel inferior because I'm not doing everything I can, I'll get stubborn. I'm not going to be shamed into action. But then maybe I'm cutting off my nose to spite my face. As I learn more and think further down the road, I find myself *doing* more. I realize that just because I can't go all the way and in every area, I still can make a sizable difference. In my mind, I may still lament that I haven't gone even further, and sometimes at night I can't sleep thinking about all the things I *haven't* changed in my life and in the lives of my children. In my actions, though, I try always to be forward-moving, to focus on the change I *am* making. I'm thrilled that my children began with organic food and therefore won't have to make that switch to it, as I did. It feels good to know that once I adapt in certain areas (say, eating and cleaning), I'm better armed to attack areas that previously seemed out of reach.

Step #7. Learn the ABCs of VOCs

In the alphabet soup of terms from environmental science, VOC—or "volatile organic compound"—is a red-letter one. That's because VOCs are the most common indoor air contaminants, present in every single home. VOCs are compounds that evaporate at room temperature and are carried through the air to our noses. Not all of them are bad—many occur naturally; for instance, trees and cows produce them—but the majority of VOCs are synthetic, emitted by cleaning supplies, pesticides, pressed wood, building materials, foam furniture, cosmetics, vinyl, air fresheners, and fuel. (Recall the term *off-gassing.*) You've doubtless heard of a couple types of common VOCs—formaldehyde and benzene. In the short term, these chemicals can make your eyes and throat hurt or, in people who are very sensitive, set off an asthma attack. In the long term, they're suspected to cause more serious health effects, including cancer.

How do you know VOCs are there? Sometimes it's obvious: They smell. Think of new carpet odor or the scent of a recently hung vinyl shower curtain—those are VOCs you're inhaling. Others, however, are odorless. We can never quite know what makes up the complex airborne stew that fills our homes, since its particular ingredients depend on what exactly in our homes is contributing to it. What are some ways to eliminate all those smells that go beyond obnoxiousness to noxiousness?

ENERGY SAVER
De-gunk your
HVAC regularly
No matter what sort of cooling/ heating system you have, change filters often to avoid mold, dust, and particle buildup. Signing up for a periodic duct-cleaning (the frequency depends on the type) can improve the efficiency of your system and help it last longer.

Take it outside. It would be great if we could all buy organic everything—wool carpets, bamboo flooring, cotton-filled furniture, etc. But if you're buying a conventionally made product that contains synthetic substances like plastic, foam, or stain repellents, then let your new purchase off-gas for a period outside. Did you order a new car seat? Take it out of the box and let it sit outdoors for a day or two (the foam inside is likely treated with flame retardants, and the plastic is made from vinyl). With carpet, request that the store or manufacturer unroll it at the warehouse to let it air out before delivery. Dry-cleaning should be removed from its plastic shroud and hung outdoors. Before use, always wash new clothing, bedding, and draperies to dissolve some of the finishing chemicals added during manufacturing.

Avoid the major triggers. Now that you're savvy to some of the health hazards of synthetic

1,000 household items, you may want to buy more con-
estimated number scientiously. Especially when looking to build a
of times worse nursery, playroom, or any place where children
indoor air is than spend lots of time, consider purchasing products
outdoor air, made of healthier materials. Start incrementally
immediately after with an organic mattress, or by using low-VOC
painting with paint, or by hanging a canvas or organic cotton
conventional paint. shower curtain rather than a vinyl one. Following
(Environmental is a list of some of the main sources of VOCs
Protection Agency, in household products. Do what you can to re-
2007) duce your exposure to these, and learn more
about healthier versions of each in the following
chapters:

- Cleaning products (Chapter 2)
- Carpets, drapes, foam-filled furniture, and mattresses (Chapter 9)
- Paints, varnishes, and lacquers (Chapter 9)
- Particleboard and other reconstituted wood (Chapter 9)
- Dry-cleaned clothing (Chapter 2)
- Plastic toys (Chapter 5)
- Air fresheners and deodorants (Chapter 2)
- Vinyl flooring and wallpaper (Chapter 9)
- Personal fragrances (Chapter 4)
- Conventional mattresses (Chapter 9)

Step #8. Install Air-Testing Devices

Some of the most insidious indoor air pollutants are odorless *and* col-
orless. How could you possibly know if your indoor air is tainted? You
can have your air professionally tested. However, simply installing inexpensive monitors is great for peace of mind and is potentially life-
saving, in the unlikely event that levels of the following hazardous
gases become dangerous.

Radon. This odorless radioactive gas occurs naturally in soil and may seep into homes, through tiny cracks in the concrete; basements are the likely place to detect radon, which is the second-leading cause of lung cancer. To test for it yourself, buy a kit at a hardware store (for around ten dollars); the test takes minutes and you'll have results in a couple days. Or, to hire a qualified radon service professional, visit epa.gov/iaq/whereyoulive.html and pick your state.

Carbon monoxide. CO, produced when any fuel (e.g., gas, fuel oil, natural gas, kerosene, wood, coal, charcoal) is burned, can accumulate rapidly indoors, and may cause headaches and dizziness, and can even be fatal within minutes. Place the monitors outside bedrooms and other areas of the home to warn you when CO (likely from the furnace, gas stove, or garage) reaches dangerous levels. Small units typically cost about forty dollars. For a more sensitive, low-level detector that indicates when carbon monoxide concentrations exceed the limit recommended by the EPA, call Multiple Chemical Sensitivity Referral and Resources, 410-362-6400.

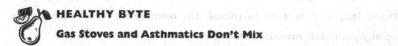

HEALTHY BYTE
Gas Stoves and Asthmatics Don't Mix

When the oven door opens, out comes nitrogen dioxide, a pollutant that can irritate breathing. A child with asthma shouldn't even be sitting in the kitchen when the oven's in use. In fact, when using a gas stove—regardless of whether there's an asthmatic in the house—crack a window or hit the vent switch.

Smoke. Obviously you'll notice it at *some* point—you just hope it's not too late. The price of smoke detectors is modest, and they should be installed outside bedrooms, basements, and also in the kitchen. In many places, it's the law. (Most insurance companies will give you a discount on your fire insurance for smoke detectors and fire extinguishers.)

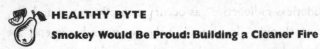

HEALTHY BYTE

Smokey Would Be Proud: Building a Cleaner Fire

Fireplaces and wood stoves can contribute mightily to indoor air problems. To offset these, burn wood that's dry, hard, solid, and plentiful.

Dry: Wood that's been "seasoned" or dried outside for at least six months burns hotter and cleaner than wood that's green (as in the color, not the philosophy).

Hard: Wood from deciduous trees, the kind that shed leaves in the fall, is harder than wood from coniferous trees, or evergreens, whose wood tends to be soft and sappy. Hardwoods such as oak, maple, hickory, apple, and ash burn hotter, longer, and cleaner than softwoods, like pine, spruce, and fir.

Solid: Never burn pressure-treated wood, particleboard, or plywood, which contain toxic chemicals such as formaldehyde and arsenic in their preservatives and adhesives. Also avoid burning plastics, newsprint, and magazines in your stove or fireplace, though you can start the fire with a bit of newsprint.

Plentiful: Once the fire's well-stoked, fill the wood stove with largeish, long-burning loads to reduce the number of times you must open the stove door or firescreen to reload, the primary means of introducing smoky pollutants into the indoor air.

A yearly chimney sweeping is recommended to remove creosote—a black tarlike or flaky deposit—which builds up on the chimney lining, blocking the exhaust of smoke and raising the risk of chimney fire.

Asbestos. A naturally occurring mineral fiber similar to fiberglass, asbestos was used in thousands of consumer products, including insulation, roofing, siding, vinyl floor tiles, and other building materials, before it was phased out in the 1970s because of health hazards associated with exposure to airborne asbestos fibers. Fibers become airborne when products containing asbestos are damaged or disturbed. If you suspect your home may be hiding asbestos—for example, if it was built between 1930 and 1950, when asbestos was frequently used for insulation—don't panic. If the structure containing the asbestos is in good condition, then the best thing is to leave it alone. However, if you want to contact a qualified professional, start your search at epa.gov/asbestos/pubs/regioncontact.html.

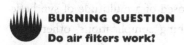

BURNING QUESTION
Do air filters work?

Air filters and purifiers may indeed pull their weight in homes with asthmatics and allergy sufferers: The EPA, at least, claims that an air filter can play a big role, along with proper ventilation and other efforts, in maintaining healthy indoor air.

High-efficiency or HEPA filters will remove particles like dust, pollen, and pet dander, while specialized charcoal-based filters can remove odors, VOC gases, chemicals, and smoke. But these are typically only strong enough to purify the air in a single room with the door closed, not a whole house.

You may also see ads for electronic purifiers, including "ion generators" that create an ionic charge to attract particles onto a collection plate, and ozone generators, which are designed to reduce the levels of some pollutants. But these have yet to prove their effectiveness, and some may even be dangerous as ozone generators have been found to create by-products that make the air *more* polluted.

In any case, no machine can do the job of the preventive measures described throughout this chapter.

Step #9. Freshen Air Naturally

Everyone's home has a different odor, and you no doubt recognize yours instantly when crossing the threshold into your house. The commingling of kitchen scents, furniture off-gassing, mold, building materials, pets, and other factors all combine to form a unique cocktail that "smells like home." So the first thing you should know is that by taking some of the precautionary measures in this chapter—ventilating well, reducing mildew and dampness, picking up piles of soggy laundry, cleaning with nontoxic supplies—your house will smell less funky, negating the need for air fresheners.

Still, you might be attached to the floral scent you get from a plug-in air freshener, or the seductive cinnamon of an aromatherapy candle or incense. Artificial fragrances are composed of a multitude of synthetic chemicals, some of which cause breathing complications, others that may cause more serious health problems. Aerosol air fresheners, meanwhile, spew tiny droplets that are easily inhaled. You're better off losing these scents and, to get your room smelling nice, doing it the natural way—with flowers, fresh air, plants, and nontoxic odor-cutters.

Bone up on fragrance labels. For scented products like cleansers and air fresheners, pick ones that contain natural or no artificial fragrances. But it can be tricky to tell what's *really* unscented. "Fragrance-free" and "no fragrance added" generally mean what they say, while "unscented" may simply mean that some synthetic chemicals were included to cover up the (bad) smell of other chemicals, yielding a more neutral scent.

Air fresheners sometimes even use nasal-numbing chemicals that trick you into "smelling" fresher air. Plus, in a Natural Resources Defense Council study of fourteen commonly available air fresheners, hormone-disrupting phthalates were found in twelve of them, some of which were labeled as "all-natural" or "unscented." For the complete list of air fresheners tested and the results, visit nrdc.org.

Burn a better candle. Candles warm a room, literally and metaphorically, but can be lousy for kids' health. For one, some candles have metal core wicks made of lead or lead-containing alloys. These candles are now banned in the United States but may still be found knocking around in drawers, and imported candles may contain them. To test yours, separate the strands of the wick to see if there's a metallic core; if the core leaves a gray mark when rubbed on white paper, it's probably got lead in it.

Also, candle wax can be a respiratory irritant. Scented candles release more chemicals (such as formaldehyde and benzene) and soot when burned than unscented ones. You can reduce soot by trimming the wick to a quarter inch and keeping the candle out of drafts. Better yet, try soy and beeswax candles, especially those that use only pure plant essential oils, which burn cleaner.

Green your air. Houseplants not only release blood-enriching oxygen, but some of them cleanse your indoor air of chemicals. A study conducted by NASA identified several houseplants that reduce the concentration of common contaminants in the air. Plus, most can flourish in low sunlight and they're easy to maintain. These are some of the best:

English ivy
Spider plant
Golden pothos or Devil's ivy
Peace lily
Chinese evergreen
Bamboo palm or Reed palm
Snake plant or Mother-in-law's tongue
Heartleaf philodendron
Selloum philodendron
Elephant ear philodendron
Red-edged dracaena
Cornstalk dracaena
Janet Craig dracaena
Warneck dracaena
Weeping fig
Gerbera daisy or Barberton daisy
Pot mum or Florist's chrysanthemum
Rubber plant

NASA's recommendation: For an 1,800-square-foot house, place fifteen to eighteen such plants in six- to eight-inch diameter containers.

Note that houseplants, including some of those listed above, may be poisonous if ingested, so take extra care with young children or pets around. Your neighborhood garden center can advise you on the non-toxic choices.

Deodorize the old-fashioned way. Some ingredients absorb and cut odors: That's how grandma no doubt kept her house cleanly scented. For a fresher whiff in the kitchen, leave coffee grounds out on the kitchen counter; in the trash can or fridge, try baking soda; and in the garbage disposal, a lemon slice. Pretty simple.

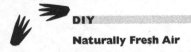

DIY

Naturally Fresh Air

Air Purifying Spritz. Love your Lysol a bit too much? Here's a natural way to dispel odors. Baking soda absorbs smells while vinegar deodorizes.

    1 teaspoon baking soda

    1 teaspoon vinegar or lemon juice

    2 cups hot water

Put all ingredients in a spray bottle and spritz in the air to kill odors.

Air Freshening Spray.

10 drops of your favorite essential oil*

7 tablespoons water

Put into a spray bottle, shake well, spray.

    * For a calming scent, try lavender; for freshness, orange and bergamot; for kitchen and bathroom, lemon and pine.

    Note: Essential oils smell so good your child may want to take a taste, so be careful—they can irritate the mouth and lungs and even be poisonous.

Step #10. Don't Run on Fumes

Many of us spend so much time commuting and driving kids around that the car has become a second home. How's the air in there? New car interiors look spectacular and smell overwhelming. Here are some ways to keep from being auto-stifled:

Open windows slightly in heavy, slow-moving traffic. Keep fresh air flowing in and reduce carbon monoxide buildup inside the car. Of course, if semis or buses in the next lane are spewing fumes into the car, it's preferable to close windows and flip on the air-conditioning.

Off-gas your new auto. The factory-fresh plastics, upholstery, carpeting, and other synthetic materials give off volatile chemicals for months afterward, so leave windows open as much as possible during that time, while driving and even when the car is parked in a (dry) garage. The less air-conditioned and recirculated air you use, the better.

Keep out engine exhaust while the car is running. Your mechanic should check yearly for air leaks into the car interior. Before starting the car after a snow, check the tailpipe for snow blockage.

Install a carbon monoxide detector in your garage. It'll ensure the gas isn't building to a dangerous level.

Expert Opinion

The Sixty-four-thousand-pound Gorilla: Your Attached Garage

By Peter L. Pfeiffer, principal of Barley and Pfeiffer Architects,
NAHB Green Advocate of the Year (2004)

The room attached to your home—the garage—harbors a variety of chemicals and substances that you want to keep out of children's reach (that's why you store them there). Half-open cans of paint, bags of fertilizers, spilled oil, car grease—these all off-gas significantly, more so as weather gets hotter or more humid. And don't forget your car, which is full of chemicals and plastics and off-gasses for hours after you park it. When you open the door to your home, there's a vacuum effect: These airborne chemicals and hydrocarbons come rushing in—especially when air ducts from air-conditioning and heating units aren't sealed tightly.

Do an air-duct seal test to ensure the duct system is functioning efficiently and this vacuum scenario doesn't occur. Ensure that the doors and access areas to the garage are well-sealed with proper weather stripping. Also, because garage walls typically lack a vapor barrier—allowing vapors to pass into the house—consider installing an exhaust fan or vents to let the garage ventilate. Finally, clean the garage of obvious culprits and always pull out immediately after turning your car on in the garage—car engines and systems these days don't need to "warm up."

 ONE STEP BEYOND
Become a Defender of Clean Air and Water

Take action on local, national, and global water and air issues by volunteering or donating to one of the many excellent nongovernment organizations devoted to the cause: Oceana, Clean Air Council, Coalition for Clean Air, Clean Air Watch, Waterkeeper's Alliance. Find out more about these in the Healthy Resources section.

CHAPTER 8

BFF

RAISING A GREEN PET

More than half of Americans have pets, the majority of them in households with children. Having a cat or dog provides huge benefits—aside from companionship and access to extensive nuzzling, of course—including greater probability of decreased blood pressure, stress, cholesterol and triglyceride levels, and increased longevity. We treat our pets as family members, so naturally we wouldn't want to put anything on them—powders, collars, sprays, and shampoos containing dangerous insecticides—that could harm them or our children. It's of special concern because kids are more likely to spend time smooching and petting the pooch or kitty, plus they roll around in places where allergens and the residue from pet products are most likely to linger.

Here are ten ways to clean up your act, and your pet's, for the sake of the family (shaggy and non-). Note: Although birds, fish, hamsters, and their ilk are common starter pets, they don't present the same issues for children's health as cats and dogs—even if you *do* kiss your guinea pig.

Step #1. Remove Allergy Triggers

Animal dander and the dust mites that feed on dander can trigger allergic reactions in humans ranging from sneezing and watery eyes to more severe breathing problems, and can aggravate asthma. To clear the air:

Vacuum regularly. Suck up clingy surfaces at least once a week—rugs, furniture, bedding, car, and anywhere else Fluffy likes to hang; more often, if your pet sheds frequently. A vacuum with a HEPA filter traps microparticles rather than blowing them back into the air.

Set boundaries. If sniffles are a problem for younger family members, designate allergy-free zones or rooms where animals aren't allowed. Keep pets outdoors as much as possible.

Lather up. Cats generally self-clean, but your dog needs weekly bathing to remove dander. Regular washing can reduce allergens by more than 80 percent—use any hypoallergenic pet shampoo. If you've run out, use a mild, nonchemical dishwashing soap rather than a mild human shampoo because the pH of the dish soap is closer to that of dogs' skin. You might want to follow up with conditioner, since shampoo can dry the skin's natural oils, generating more dander. Find safe, eco-friendly grooming supplies at holistic pet stores and online (see Healthy Resources).

Wash your own paws. After playing with pets, family members should wash hands thoroughly with soap and water, especially before scratching skin or touching eyes.

Pick pet-friendly furnishings. Cloth curtains, horizontal blinds, and carpeted floors tend to trap animal dander and other allergy-causing particles. Minimize surfaces that harbor these triggers.

Purify the air. Install a HEPA filter to prevent dander from recirculating throughout the home. Put them over vents and change seasonally. (For more on air filters, see Chapter 7.)

Check for red herrings. If a person reacts to animal allergens, he or she may be allergic to other substances in the house: dust mites, mold, soaps, pesticides, mildew, and feathers. Clean up these other irritating particles; Mr. Biggles may not be the only culprit.

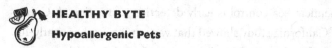

HEALTHY BYTE
Hypoallergenic Pets

Some breeds produce fewer allergens because they shed less or lack a gene that creates a certain protein. Dogs that shed minimally and don't leave dander include the Labradoodle, poodle, bichon frise, and Wheaton terrier; among cat breeds, the Sphynx and Devon rex are kinder to allergy sufferers.

Step #2. Make Fleas Flee, Naturally

When pesky fleas hop a ride on a pooch or kitty, pet owners often rush out to buy sprays, flea collars, powders, foggers, and bombs, or have the vet dunk the animal in flea repellent. It wasn't until 1996 that the EPA started to examine the risks of pet pesticide products; even today, the agency's toxicity testing is far from thorough. But pesticides can make your pets sick, and can be unhealthy for everyone else in your family, too. Pregnant women should absolutely avoid contact with these chemicals.

HEALTHY BYTE
Unsafe Pet Pest Products

Pesticides, like those in pet products, aren't thoroughly regulated for health by the government. The following ingredients have been shown in lab tests to be health risks; if you see them on the label of flea and tick collars or bombs, steer clear.

Organophosphates (OPs). Chlorpyrifos; Dichlorvos; Phosmet; Naled; Tetrachlorvinphos; Diazinon; Malthion.

Carbamates. Carbaryl; Propoxur.

Deflea your home the nontoxic way. Within eight hours of a flea laying eggs on your cat or dog, about 70 percent of the eggs will have fallen onto the carpet or the pet's bedding, where the larvae thrive. To eliminate them without resorting to chemicals:

- **Vacuum early and often.** The single most effective weapon in nonchemical flea control is early detection and action. A University of California study showed that vacuuming catches nearly 100 percent of adult fleas. Plus, vacuuming may help to shake eggs and larvae from carpeting and bedding. If there's an infestation, vacuum daily; after cleaning, seal the vacuum bag inside a plastic trash bag and discard. Vacuum the car or furniture your pet frequents.

- **Wash bedding.** Since immature fleas don't tend to hang out on their host, regularly laundering doggie bed covers can help reduce proliferation. Better still, replace the bed with a cedar-filled one, which repels fleas, and has removable covers (but beware that cedar can trigger asthma in some kids). When fleas are especially invasive, wash bedding and throw rugs once or twice weekly.

- **Use a flea trap.** These employ an incandescent lightbulb to attract fleas, which are then trapped on sticky paper. A nonmanufacturer study found traps effective at capturing 10 percent of adult fleas; studies sponsored by trap makers found they're up to 95 percent effective. Disparity aside, traps, coupled with other nonpesticide methods, are worth trying.

- **Try the white socks and water trick.** Seriously. Don white socks and put a few bowls of water around the room where you want to eradicate fleas. Shuffle around the floor slowly and the hungry fleas will feel your heat and jump on the socks. Pick them off or hold the sock right over the water and dunk to drown the fleas.

- **Nominate nematodes.** Nema-what? They're tiny worms you embed in your garden or lawn to infect and kill flea larvae. They can eliminate 90-plus percent of larvae in the first twenty-four hours.

Apply them to the soil in areas where your pet digs and buries whatever it is he buries. Nematodes need about 20 percent soil moisture to survive, so water the area every few days. They're sold through pet stores and garden suppliers.

🌀 Expert Opinion 🌀
My Best Advice
By Dr. Jeffrey Werber, veterinarian (and Lassie's vet)

I became a veterinarian because as a kid I just loved dogs and cats. Their playful innocence is not unlike that of children, whose curiosity can expose them to harm.

One of the concerns that veterinarians face today is the use of pesticides on pets—and whether or not they pose a risk, not only to the pet but to the child that may be in close association with the animal when the application is administered. The danger to children from pesticides on pets comes from two sources. One is the application to the animal. The other is when the animals pick up pesticides from the environment, like those applied to lawns. In both cases, children can be directly exposed to the pesticide by touching the pet and also by the pesticide coming in contact with the home environment, on the floors and in the carpet where small children and especially toddlers like to play.

My best advice to eradicate fleas in a more natural manner is to use many of the practical, nontoxic suggestions offered in this chapter. By keeping your pets' home environment clean, giving frequent baths (dogs are easier than cats) and using a good flea comb—this should help to ensure a safer environment for both your children and your pets.

To deal with fleas on the pet (the other 30 percent):
- **Feed them brewer's yeast.** Extra vitamin B, like that in brewer's (not baker's) yeast, makes animals less tasty to fleas. For cats, sprinkle a half to one teaspoonful of yeast daily on food; for big dogs, try a quarter cup of yeast, less for smaller dogs. Or, under the supervision of your vet, choose a B-vitamin complex pill.

- **Comb out pests.** A fine-tooth metal flea comb is an effective, pesticide-free way to catch fleas or at least force them to jump off Snuffles. Comb them outside, with a ready container of soapy water to drown the fleas; or do it in a bathtub where you can rinse pests down the drain. After running the comb gently through your pet's coat, dunk it in the water and wriggle any fur caught in the comb into the soapy water, killing the fleas. Do this for your pet's whole body. During a severe infestation, repeat daily.

- **Give a clean bath.** Pesticide shampoos are unnecessary. Soap kills fleas, if left on for five to eight minutes. If dry skin is a concern, avoid dander by sometimes using conditioner alone.

- **Use natural flea collars and sprays.** These will be easily identifiable as "nontoxic" or "herbal" collars and contain varying combinations of eucalyptus, citronella, rosemary, lemongrass, cedar, sesame, and natural fragrances. The herbs don't kill fleas but can repel them (keep fragrant oils away from kids, who may ingest them). Plus, they probably smell nicer than the "poison necklaces" of chemical flea collars.

  96
  percentage of adult fleas wiped out by regular vacuuming.
  (Journal of Economic Entomology, 1986)

  - **Try antiflea sachets.** Fill envelopes with lavender, mint, rosemary, sweet woodruff, or cedar, and stuff them between couch cushions. Fleas hate the scents.

 DIY

Doggie Flea Repellents

Spritz. Citrus oil kills and repels fleas. Place four cut lemons in a saucepan and cover with water. Bring to a boil and simmer for fifteen minutes. Cool, then strain the liquid into a glass container. Apply liquid liberally to fur, while brushing, so oil penetrates the skin. Dry with a towel and brush again.

   Sprinkle. Mix a half cup baking soda and a half teaspoon orange oil. Blend. Dust onto your pet and work into the fur.

Step #3. Solve Your #2 Problem

Not only is animal waste unsightly and stinky, it transmits disease and parasites to people. Two intestinal parasites, ascarids and hookworms, are common in puppies and kittens; the CDC has determined that eating dirt is the primary way of contracting these parasites. Since children are prone to licking dirt from their hands after playing outside, they're more vulnerable than adults.

But that's not the only way animal excrement affects kids. When owners don't pick up after their pets, the waste is washed down into the sewage systems, then into nearby lakes and rivers your children wade and swim in. Dog waste is a significant contributor to bacteria in waterways.

Use biodegradable doggie bags, so your pooch's deposit won't stay contained in a landfill for centuries. Biobagusa.com sells biodegradable dog and cat poop bags made from genetically unmodified corn, and claims their bags biodegrade at the same rate as an apple.

Avoid clumping and clay kitty litters. Clay is strip-mined and filled with silica dust that may irritate your cat's—and child's—lungs. The clumping agent, sodium bentonite (used also in grouting, sealing, and plugging agents), can swell up to eighteen times its dry size and poison your cat if it eats enough. Safer cat litters aren't loaded with clay and chemicals to clump and control odor. Green pet stores carry varieties like 100 percent all-natural wood, (nonfood grade) wheat, biodegradable paper, and corn mixtures, all of which rapidly break down and dissolve.

Pregnant women should not handle litter boxes. Toxoplasmosis, a potentially serious disease that can infect the fetus and cause birth defects or miscarriage, is transmitted through cat feces. Women who are expecting should stay away from litter boxes and outdoor areas where cats have pooped, avoid handling stray cats, and never feed cats undercooked or raw meat. Wash hands thoroughly with soap and running water after playing with animals, and be especially careful to avoid cat scratches and bites.

Parentblog
The Bugs Aren't the Real Problem
By Tessa Hill, president of Kids
for Saving Earth

I grew up in Minnesota, where we generally didn't use pesticides in our homes. Then, when I was twenty-seven, my husband and I moved to Houston, Texas. I was shocked at the number of fleas and roaches in our new home and yard. The natives said it was customary to spray your house four times a year. The exterminator sprayed kitchen countertops, baseboards, bathrooms—everyplace. When I expressed concern, he said, *Don't worry; we'll use something without an odor.*

A few years later, there was an infestation of lice at my son's school. Clint was one of those who got it, and the nurse called to have me take him home. She gave me a long list of what to do. I think it's natural to feel panicky, and I didn't want him to miss school, so I did what I was told: applied the lice medication she recommended, washed bedding and towels, and sprayed carpet, furniture, car seats, etc., with aerosol lice medication. A few weeks later, Clint got lice again and we went through the whole chemical process once more.

Sadly, I had no idea that lice medications can contain pesticides. As instructed, I placed it directly on Clint's head. Now I ask, *Why would anyone think pesticides wouldn't also harm or even kill humans?*

Six months later, Clint was diagnosed with a malignant brain tumor. He was in unbearable pain. Before we could catch our breath, we were in the hospital, for surgery to remove a baseball-sized tumor.

Many scientists believe that an individual may have a genetic predisposition or weakness to cancer, and when your immunity is being pummeled—say, by chemicals all around you, in your home, food, yard, the air—it saps your cancer-fighting strength. Some people can smoke for years but have the genes to fight off cancer.

In the hospital I saw lots of children with cancer. We were asked numerous times about our genetic background but not once about our environmental background. I suggest hospitals keep records about environmental exposure.

Clinton was eleven when he died. I don't know for sure if pesticides caused his death. Many scientific studies suggest a link between pesticides and brain cancer. I do know that it isn't worth taking a chance with toxic bug control methods. There are many safe ways to eradicate pests, including lice. I used boric acid to beat back a roach infestation at our beach house; it worked beautifully and didn't contaminate the property. I refuse to use standard mosquito sprays or flea treatments that contain cancer-causing chemicals.

Before he died, Clint wanted to start a club to teach kids and parents about environmental issues. Kids for Saving Earth (kidsforsavingearth.org), which provides materials to educate and empower children, parents, and instructors about ways to protect the Earth and children's environmental health, is Clint's legacy.

Step #4. Feed Your Pets Healthy Foods

Decades ago, a dog or cat would simply have eaten scraps off its owner's table (and probably supplemented its meals with mice, birds, and other entrees from nature). But today's pets dine on many of the same pesticide- and preservative-laden foods that we do. Conventional pet foods are even worse: The main source of protein in both dry and canned food is "down animals"—creatures brought to the slaughter-house because they're one of the "four D's" (disabled, diseased, dying, or dead)—or low-grade waste products such as cartilage and bones.

The conventional pet diet, which is overprocessed and low in nutrients—despite all sorts of claims about its being "scientifically balanced"—has triggered a jump in pet diseases now common in humans, including diabetes and allergies. Given the unpronounceable ingredients in pet food, you wouldn't want your curious toddler to wonder what her cat's lunch tastes like.

Look for real food on labels. A label that starts with "beef" or "liver" is superior to one that begins with "by-product," "by-product meal," "meat and bone meal," or "meat." Choose foods that are tagged with Association of American Feed Control Officials (AAFCO) standards for complete and balanced nutrition. The label also means that no animal testing was performed.

Switch to wheat gluten–free foods. Doing so may also ease your mind, considering the large-scale 2007 Chinese pet food recall, in which it appears that melamine-tainted wheat gluten resulted in the deaths of numerous dogs and cats. Additive- and grain-free brands tend to be purer.

Introduce fresh foods. You needn't feed your pet organic foie gras; just supplement his diet with healthy fresh foods—proteins such as beef, chicken, salmon, turkey, and eggs, and lots of fresh and steamed veggies and fruits (avoid onions, grapes, avocados, and raisins, which are hard for animals to digest and can be harmful). Use in equal proportions: one-third meat, one-third fruit/vegetable, one-third healthy grains (grains should be cooked and cereals presoaked to soften them). It's ideal for pet digestion if you grind it all up in a food processor or blender. If your pet needs help digesting some foods, consult your vet about getting supplemental digestive enzymes.

One healthy snack your dog will love: a marrow bone that you can buy at the butcher or meat counter at the supermarket. It keeps him occupied for hours and is good for teeth.

Provide clean pet water. For pets kept outdoors or dogs that go on hikes, drinking runoff water may cause giardia, a microbe that's very contagious among humans (and can be transmitted from dogs to humans). Bring a fresh source of drinking water with you. If your pet spends time in the yard, keep a bowl outside.

Also, pets are likely as susceptible to impurities in tap water—lead and other metals, arsenic, microbes—as we are, so if your family drinks from a filtered container or tap, don't assume unfiltered water is just fine for your dog or cat. To minimize microbial growth, change water bowls daily, especially if there's a curious toddler nearby.

In the long run, feeding your pet a healthier diet can save on vet bills. And heartier pets are more likely to fight off irritating or dangerous pests.

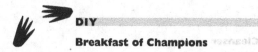

DIY

Breakfast of Champions

This recipe will get your pooch off to an energetic start.

½ cup brown rice

2 cups chopped mixed veggies (cauliflower, broccoli, carrots)

1 cup ground organic chicken/turkey/lamb

½ cup uncooked oats

3 cage-free omega-3 eggs

1 cup fat-free plain yogurt

1 cup chicken or beef broth

½ cup water with 1 chicken stock cube dissolved

Cook the rice and put it in a medium-size casserole or pie dish with the vegetables, chicken, and oats. Mix well.

In a bowl, beat together the eggs, yogurt, and broth. Fold the egg mixture into the rice mixture. Cook in the oven at 375°F for 30 minutes, or until set.

Cut into wedges and serve. (Unused portions can be frozen.)

—*from: Tamar Geller, author of* The Loved Dog: The Playful, Non-Aggressive Way to Teach Your Dog Good Behavior

Step #5. Give a Better Bath

Shampoo your pooch on a regular basis with gentle, nontoxic shampoos and/or conditioners. Again, it's better for your pet, and healthier for kids who like to bury their face in fur. If washing your pet is something you do outside, nontoxic products are better for the Earth (when I was a kid, my mom used to toss us a bottle of Prell and we'd shampoo our dog in the stream behind the house—whoops). Safe suds include organic baby shampoo, Castile or nontoxic oil soap, or herbal shampoos and conditioners that contain essential-oil repellents.

DIY

Nontoxic Pet Cleanser

¼ teaspoon essential oil repellent (citronella, cedarwood, eucalyptus, rosemary, or bay leaf)

1 teaspoon mild shampoo (Castile or other chemical-free type)

1 cup water

Mix thoroughly, pour over pet, and massage into its coat, making sure to avoid its eyes and mouth. Let the solution dry out a bit before rinsing. If your pet is extra-sensitive to essential oils, decrease the amount applied.

Step #6. Fetch Healthy Toys

Dogs use their mouths to carry everything, so make sure that what he's chewing won't hurt him. Then, of course, kids pick up and play with pets' toys—and a teething baby may confuse her cat's squeaky rubber mouse for her own. Instead of a plastic squeeze or chew toy, which may contain hormone-disrupting phthalates, opt for toys made from rawhide, wool, hemp, natural rubber, or any chemical-free fibers. Make sure these toys don't come with buttons or other small pieces that pets can swallow. You can also turn old clothing into fun toys. Cut strips from mangled scarves, unsalvageable sweaters, or unused knitting yarn, then tie together . . . voilà! Your chew-happy pup has something to munch on (and has helped you to declutter, too).

✺ Expert Opinion ✺
Nature's Pet
By Tamar Geller, author of The Loved Dog: The Playful,
Non-Aggressive Way to Teach Your Dog Good Behavior

Dogs are the amazing bridge between nature and ourselves. Every dog's psychodynamic is a little bit like a wolf and a little bit like a toddler. As dog owners, we have to celebrate our similarity, which is the toddler part, and our difference, which is the wolf part.

Kids and dogs have a lot of the same needs. They have the need for certainty: of knowing that they are loved and have a home, that they have a reliable leader who is there to teach them with kindness. And they have the need for secure attachment, the reassurance that they're connected to someone, like a toddler at the playground who keeps looking back at his mommy. One of the big similarities is the need for playing games.

One game I encourage is tug-of-war. It's a misunderstood game, as people think that it will encourage aggression in their dog. But played right, it will put you in a position of being the leader while strengthening your relationship with your dog. In nature, this is the game that tells us which one of us will end up with the piece of meat (and therefore is higher in the pecking order). At home, if you end up with the plush squeaky toy, you position *yourself* as the leader. (I recommend one made of organic materials with a squeaker inside.) You are also giving your dog an outlet for his wolf energy in a constructive way, and you become the leader of the pack by playing it right: The dog looks at you and thinks, *Wow, I'm understood!* A few keys to the game: The owner must be the one to start and finish the game; he should be able to ask the dog to "drop" the toy and have the dog comply (use treats); he should finish the game while the dog's interest is still high; and he should take the toy with him.

When a dog feels that both his toddler and his wolf needs are being met, that he matters, then you'll have a happy, secure, well-mannered dog. That's what I try to teach people: that good dog coaching means giving it a level of respect and appreciation for nature—celebrate the nature of the wolf that is in your dog. Isn't that what living green is all about? Living an examined life, and recognizing that every choice you make has consequences to your world.

Step #7. Let Sleeping Dogs Lie ... in a Green Bed

Yes, even Fido and Fifi can rest easy on an organic mattress. Made with organic cotton (free from synthetic dyes), hemp, or other fiber, and stuffed with natural filling like organically grown buckwheat hulls, green pet beds won't release pet-unfriendly fumes like foam beds do. You can also find hemp collars and leashes and recycled cardboard cat trees.

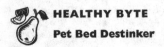 **HEALTHY BYTE**
Pet Bed Destinker

Sprinkle baking soda on the bed, leave it for an hour or more, then shake it off.

Another healthy accoutrement: Rather than plastic bowls, which can leach chemicals into your pet's food and water, use stainless steel bowls. Ceramic is also safe, but more breakable, especially with kids around.

Step #8. Clean Up Your Pet's Turf

Like us, pets are extremely sensitive to chemicals in lawn products. They may ingest excessive amounts when they lick their paws, and some actually like to eat grass. Dogs exposed to fertilizers and some herbicides have been found to have unusually high levels of heavy metals in their blood, and some studies have linked lawn chemicals to bladder cancer and lymphoma in canines. Several lawn chemicals come in pellet form and look an awful lot like dog food; as a result, many dogs have been poisoned. If you must use chemicals, keep these products tightly sealed in your garage and store them on a high shelf or in a locked cabinet. Other products that tempt (and harm) animals include fertilizer sprays (particularly toxic to cats), rat poison, and antifreeze.

For the safety of your whole extended family, green your lawn using organic, nonchemical techniques. (For information on how to do that, see Chapter 6.)

Driveway deicing products are also hazardous to dogs. Chloride salts, the most common deicer, irritate the skin of pets and can even poison them if they lick their feet. Avoid carbonyl diamide—a.k.a. urea—to melt ice: It releases nitrate when it enters the water supply, causing algae blooms.

In winter, if you're worried about traction on your driveway and walkway, spread sand and gravel instead of a chemical product. If you sweep it up for reuse, their environmental impact will be minimal. Or try pet-, child-, and environmentally harmless Safe Paw.

Finally, pets that spend time outside will track in everything they contact, including pesticides, feces, and other contaminants. Wipe your pooch's paws with a wet rag or sponge.

Step #9. Fur Sure

As mentioned, shampoos can be overly drying for some animals' skin, contributing to a dander problem, in which case you should opt occasionally for chemical-free conditioners.

If your pet seems to have irritated skin, hot or raw spots, or is constantly licking her feet, it could be an allergic reaction to something in her diet. A home-cooked meal, with supplements to help your pet digest, is the best way to minimize allergic reactions. (See Step #4 for pet food tips.) When in doubt, seek advice from your veterinarian.

To treat skin irritations, many green pet experts swear by natural treatments such as coconut oil and raw honey, which you can give internally or use as a salve.

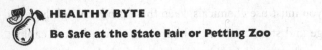

HEALTHY BYTE
Be Safe at the State Fair or Petting Zoo

Fair and zoo exhibits allow kids to explore all sorts of animals, from watching bare bronc riding at a rodeo to feeding goats at a county fair. But this interaction also puts young children at risk for contracting E. coli from cows and calves, and salmonella from chickens and turtles. To reduce risk:

Wash hands. Locate hand-washing stations. Wash your hands and your children's hands after petting any animals or even touching the animal's cage or fence, buckets, bedding, and especially manure.

Separate food. Keep your own food and drinks clear of animal areas. Don't allow children to share their funnel cake, cotton candy, or any other food with the animals. Avoid drinking any unpasteurized dairy products.

Supervise children. Kids under five need to be watched so they won't put their hands or objects (pacifier or bottle) in their mouths around animals or kiss animals. The CDC recommends that infants and toddlers avoid contact with reptiles, amphibians, baby chicks, ducklings, and petting zoos.

Step #10. Petcycle

Sure, purebred French bulldogs are gorgeous creatures, but unless you aim to parade them at the Westminster Dog Show, how about bringing into the family a nonpedigreed companion from a local animal shelter? Aside from the pleasure of taking in one of the grateful, formerly homeless mutts and cats who would otherwise be euthanized (the fate of 3 to 4 million of them annually) and the benefit of saving lots of money (it can cost over a thousand dollars just to buy a pure breed), there are other reasons to forego purebloods: Some breeders raise large quantities of such animals for profit (called "puppy mills"), and have been denounced by animal activists for overbreeding and inbreeding; and purebred dogs are more likely to carry genetic diseases, from epilepsy to cataracts. Mixed breeds (including today's popular "couture dogs"—

Labradoodles, cockapoos, puggles) share a bigger gene pool, and are generally healthier creatures.

Adopting an adult dog offers other pluses: Puppies may pass the bacterium *Campylobacter* and a variety of other parasites, which can cause diarrhea and rashes or illness in humans, especially among children under five. If you're still set on a certain pedigree, one-quarter of the dogs in shelters are purebred, and every breed has a rescue club. My experience is that kids don't care if it's a Maltese or a mutt, as long as it licks off their faces with love. Petfinder.com helps find local pets to rescue, purebreds and mutts alike.

 ONE STEP BEYOND

Grow your own catnip. Dazzle your feline with a taste of your own organic catnip, which may be grown indoors. Check out citycats.biz to order.

Turn poop to power. Start a program, like San Francisco's, to convert pet waste into energy. There, pet owners use biodegradable bags provided at the local dog-walk park, make deposits in special carts dubbed "methane digesters," inside of which bacteria transform the waste into methane, and which may then be used to power appliances that use natural gas. Launch that, and no one can accuse you of dogging it.

CHAPTER 9

Safe House

HEALTHY HOME IMPROVEMENT

'm a sucker for home improvement shows—they get me psyched to whip out my tools to install shelving or change every light fixture in the house. But this televised Do-It-Yourself craze has meant, more than ever, that home is not an endpoint but a work in progress. You change the paint color in the living room, redecorate the kids' bedrooms, replace the tacky old kitchen cabinetry, retile the bathroom, build a deck . . . and oh, look: time to paint the living room again.

Some people like to do things themselves; others hand it off to the pros. Either way, home improvements made for aesthetics, comfort, efficiency, sanity, and keeping-up-with-the-Joneses afford a chance to make the home healthier, too. The types of materials you bring in, from furniture to insulation to flooring to paints to linens, can variously improve indoor air quality, lower utility bills, and grant you a true sense of home sweet home.

This chapter starts with small changes that provide significant payoff, and moves toward issues to keep in mind for larger-scale overhauls. And for those interested in a down-to-the-studs renovation using healthy and green building materials, I'll point you toward some useful resources.

Step #1. Sleep Easy

We spend roughly a third of our lives asleep, so it's a no-brainer that we should do it on something that isn't bad for us. Start with a mattress made of natural material, like organic cotton, wool, or some combination of these. Ever wonder why mattresses come with those tags threatening lockup should you dare remove them? The tag certifies that a mattress is up to fire code, meaning it's covered in toxic flame retardants and other chemicals. Unlike conventional mattresses, which are made of polyurethane foam that disintegrates over time, releasing tiny particles associated with upper respiratory problems, organic mattresses are free of synthetics, including flame retardants and water repellents. You can also find mattresses made of natural latex, which deters dust mites and bacteria, and is stain- and waterproof. Note that latex can be sensitizing for people with allergies and can even trigger nut allergies; avoid them if your family has a history of these.

And the flammability issue? Wool, it happens, is a naturally flame-resistant material, and meets Consumer Product Safety Commission standards.

Natural fiber and organic mattresses do cost a lot—$1,000 to $5,000—but they last a long time: Most green manufacturers guarantee at least twenty years. If it's too expensive, prioritize: Start with a natural crib mattress, since at the beginning your baby sleeps fourteen to sixteen hours a day or even more. These start at around $250. A twin-size for a child starts at around $500.

Mattress pads. If you're not ready to splurge on an organic mattress, you can still make a difference to your child's exposure by placing an organic (and naturally flame-retardant) wool pad on the bed. Wool naturally wicks away moisture, making it a great choice for kids' beds, which are going to get peed on. Don't put down a squishy mattress pad for babies under one year because it can present a heightened SIDS risk.

Bedding. Look for sets made from unbleached, untreated organic cotton or other eco-friendly natural fibers like linen, hemp, and bamboo. Sheets, blankets, bedspreads, and comforters of any material are likely to carry chemical permanent-press, stain-repellent, and water-repellent finishes. Organic- and natural-fabric sheets come in a range of picky-taste-pleasing colors and patterns made from nontoxic dyes. If you do decide to stick with conventional bedding, wash new sheets before putting them on your bed to rinse away manufacturing residues.

Pillows. Go for natural fills, such as wool, kapok, buckwheat (which prohibit the growth of dust mites), or organic cotton. Conventional pillows are often stuffed with polyester and treated with chemical finishes (do you really want to press your face into that?). Feathers can be triggers for asthma and allergies. Use pillow encasements from an allergy product store to reduce the inhalation of dust mites.

Expert Opinion
Health Risks of Fire Retardants
By Russell Long, vice president and board member of
Friends of the Earth

Over the past three decades-plus, hundreds of millions of pounds of brominated and chlorinated fire-retardant chemicals have been put into furniture, carpets, and other products with which we have intimate daily contact. Now, virtually every American tested has been found to have some of these fire retardants stored in their bodies, with babies showing the highest levels.

Babies are especially vulnerable because they crawl or climb on furniture and carpeting treated with these chemicals, orally ingesting or inhaling them. Babies also absorb these compounds from their mothers' breast milk and through the placenta. According to scientists, North American women have some of the highest levels, nearly ten times those found in European and Asian women's breast milk. The chemicals detected include previously banned substances such as PBDEs, and those still lawfully produced, such as decaBDE.

This is especially troubling in light of recent studies that link fire-retardant exposure to cancer, birth defects, autism, thyroid disorders, hyperactivity, learning disabilities such as attention deficit disorder, and a host of other problems.

Fortunately, there is good news. Many furniture and carpet companies make smolder-resistant products free of these chemicals. Most of these use polyester fabric blends resistant to short-duration heat exposure. Even cotton, rayon, and linen, which do not resist fires, can be made fire resistant by using a 30 percent weave of polyester fibers.

In addition, twenty-two states have passed fire-safe cigarette laws that call for cigarettes that self-extinguish within five minutes, and other states are expected to follow. Because the majority of home fires start from cigarettes, these laws should substantially reduce fire risk in homes. Additionally, a number of cigarette companies have already switched to fire-safe cigarettes.

To avoid toxic chemical exposure, consumers need to ask retailers whether that new sofa, chair, carpet, or drapery contains any fire-retardant chemicals. Sometimes this is easy to figure out by looking at the labels underneath a new couch or carpet. If the label mentions flammability standards, chances are that chemicals were used. And if the retailer has no answer, consider going elsewhere. Numerous innovative manufacturers use greener chemicals or naturally fire-resistant lining such as wool, denser foams, or internal fire barriers in their "green" lines.

Addressing fire safety shouldn't come at the expense of poisoning our children and environment, especially when good alternatives exist.

Parentblog
Once Upon a Mattress
By Laura Dern, actress

We hear the news that we're having a baby and we want to be really healthy and careful. So we eat organically, avoid mercury in fish, don't drink, don't smoke; we don't use hair color or paint our nails. We spend all this energy and time creating a really healthy environment—and then we totally switch gears. We stop thinking about health and somehow lead ourselves to believe that the most important thing for the baby when it comes home from the hospital is...a pretty room. Suddenly we assume the baby's going to see its room and say, *Ugh, I hate ducks, what was she thinking?... I'm a boy, how dare she paint my room peach?* And so we choose the coolest crib design, instead of the safest or healthiest crib. We pick the absolute cutest linens, even if they're covered in flame-retardants and other chemicals (never mind that a baby can hardly see at first). Unwittingly we put loads of toxic chemicals into the room as we strive to make it look just right.

But think about it: A newborn baby is spending something like sixteen hours a day asleep. And that newborn baby's face is pressed against that space, breathing in what is probably a fresh-off-the-conveyer-belt mattress whose off-gassing is at its height. On top of that you put a bleached, chemically treated cotton sheet that's newly dyed—oh, but it's really cute!—and perhaps not even washed first, or washed in a conventional detergent that's high in chemicals. Then there's the crib itself, which is often made of particle board, and which continues to off-gas for a long time. Unbeknown to you, you've created an environment with risks when all you wanted to do was make your baby happy and safe. But it *looks* good. Even though the kid is not going to enjoy it for the first two years of his life.

Most of us do it because nobody told us not to.

That's why my gift to close friends when they have a baby is an organic or natural-fiber mattress. (If you already own a conventional mattress, there are things you can do to make it healthier, like getting organic wool and cotton pee-pee pads, instead of the plastic ones.) I encourage them to get a sustainable hardwood crib, too. They're beautiful—mine is naturally stained and waxed and looks like an old arts-and-crafts crib—and often cost no more than ordinary ones.

As parents, we can be fearful of everything from melting polar caps to which sleep strategy works best. And everyone's read every book, so most parents live in abject terror, feeling like everything is out of their control. But what we *do* control is our home environment, which is an incredible gift. We can create a wonderful safe haven for our babies, even literally within just a few square inches.

Step #2. Lose the Carpet

Considering that children spend so much time sprawled on and crawling across the floor, what's underfoot can have a vital influence on their health. Conventional carpets give off fumes from things like stainproofing and glues that can contribute to headaches and breathing problems—and may even have long-term health consequences. Also, all carpets harbor dust and allergenic bits (pet dander, fungal spores, bacteria, mold, mildew, and dust-mite droppings), as well as chemicals like pesticides tracked in from outdoors. Even the most ardent vacuuming enthusiast is challenged to keep up with rug cleaning—and conventional cleaners are brewed with extremely nasty chemicals.

Hard surface flooring—many types, anyway—is much better for your family. But if you love the softness of pile underfoot, there are healthy ways to get that, too.

A plug for rugs. Natural-fiber rugs made from pesticide-free wool, cotton, jute, hemp, coir, corn husk, coconut fiber, high-end woven silk, and other natural materials are easy to remove for cleaning and can be taken outside to air in the sun. They provide warmth and sound control and make playing on hard floors more comfortable. A vintage area rug is another good option, since old wool or oriental-type rugs were likely made without synthetics.

The best rug pads are made of untreated wool or camel's hair felt. If you can, skip pads derived from synthetic foams, foam rubber, or plastic underlays.

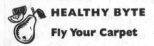

HEALTHY BYTE
Fly Your Carpet

If you're buying a conventionally made rug or carpet, ask the company or store to air it out in its warehouse for at least three days prior to installation. For at least three days *after* installation, open windows to disperse chemical fumes from the synthetic materials. Plan B: When the carpet's delivered, unroll it and store it for a week in the garage (preferably with the roll-top open) or on a covered back porch.

Pile on. If you really covet wall-to-wall, buy carpet made from natural fibers such as organic wool and made with undyed or vegetable-dyed fibers and no chemical finishes. Tack down carpets rather than gluing, or use water-based adhesives.

Another versatile, design-conscious option: carpet tiles, especially colorful ones such as those from Flor, which are made from recycled and renewable materials and emit few pollutants. These tiles can be arranged to form an area rug or laid out to cover a room; they require no glue; and because they lift up by section, it's far easier to clean stains, negating the need for nasty chemicals.

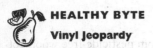

HEALTHY BYTE
Vinyl Jeopardy

As bad as synthetic carpet is, it may meet its match in vinyl flooring, made of PVC, which off-gases chemicals like formaldehyde. However, vinyl flooring that's been in your house for years is probably okay, since the fumes given off by the vinyl diminish over time.

Get a floor plan. If you're over your carpet, there are several nontoxic, hard flooring options to consider:

- **Hardwood floors.** The best material for those with allergies or chemical sensitivities, hardwood is easy to clean with a broom or vacuum and mild cleanser. However, buying new wood contributes to deforestation; the greenest choice comes from acreage managed under the guidelines of the Forest Stewardship Council (FSC), an international nonprofit dedicated to responsible caretaking of the world's forests. Another green choice: reusing reclaimed and salvaged wood from barns or tear-downs. Many regional companies specialize in salvaging old hardwoods from old buildings and homes.

    To preserve the hardwood floor that's under the carpet you're ripping up—or to refinish old planks or parquet—use water-based varnish rather than a conventional polyurethane.

- **Bamboo.** The crown prince of green design materials, bamboo, is a super alternative to conventional wood flooring: It's durable, harder than most hardwood flooring, often cheaper, and rapidly renewable (it takes only four years from planting to harvest). Almost all of it is grown without pesticides, thanks to its natural antifungal and antibacterial properties. However, make sure that whoever lays it down doesn't glue it with toxic adhesives.

    Be aware that most bamboo comes from China, so you have to consider whether you want to buy material that requires shipping halfway around the world. Where possible, use more locally sourced bamboo.

- **Cork.** Made from the inner bark of the Mediterranean cork oak, cork can be cut repeatedly from very old trees. It's composed of tiny air pockets that make the surface springy underfoot (a forgiving surface for kids); it's also hypoallergenic, and with its low-static surface is resistant to dust and pet hair. The planks or tiles are relatively easy to install, and don't require glue.

- **Natural linoleum.** Not to be mistaken for vinyl linoleum, natural linoleum is made of sawdust, linseed oil, pigments, and jute backing, and it's water- and pet stain–resistant. It's easy to put down in tiles, using nontoxic glues.

- **Tile.** Made from ceramic, stone, or recycled glass, tile is virtually VOC-free, highly durable, and easily cleaned.

And believe it or not, even *concrete* is a green option (mix in a reusable waste by-product called fly ash and it's greener still), as well as strong, handsome, easy to work with, and inexpensive.

Parentblog
I Can Look My Trees in the Eye
By Jenna Elfman, actress

Before I had a child, I'd hear people talking about green this or that, but most of it didn't seem to apply to me. I'd tell myself to try and remember something for the future—*There's chemicals in your face cream, Don't paint your walls with regular paint*—but mostly I was a lost cause. Except for recycling. I'm *obsessed* with recycling, and putting all the garbage in its own separate bins. I love to go on the Bureau of Sanitation site and...well, that's another story.

To change, you need to be willing. If it makes sense, if I can see how something applies to my life, then I'm willing to change. Eventually, of course, these issues started to apply to me. I got pregnant and had my son. I learned that installing carpet, with its glues and padding and fire retardants, and all the things that get trapped in it like lead and pesticides and dirt, was not the healthiest option. Who wants that? So now I have no carpet. I have travertine stone floors, cork floors, bamboo floors. There's a gradient scale of willingness, knowledge, and responsibility. I take it step by step.

I start with little things I can face easily. Right now I'm about to research what plastics to use (and not) for food storage. I just need twenty minutes on Google every so often. I also have organic food delivered and I switched to Seventh Generation cleaning products. (I've never liked the smell of cleaning products; but when I was pregnant, I *really* hated it.) I also use phthalate-free nail polish (that was pregnancy, too—one whiff of the regular stuff and I nearly passed out, plus it's bad for you when you're expecting). I've bought lots of organic products for the baby—crib mattress, fitted sheets, towels, sleeping gowns, clothes. I even stopped using deodorant and switched to The Rock. *Seriously.* See, there's that gradient scale again. Suddenly it all made sense. I was willing to change.

Then there are things I won't (or have yet to) do: I tried the natural toothpaste thing but that's not happening for me. I could easily use organic shampoos and face products but I don't, not yet. For now I'm sticking with what's worked for me all these years. Oh, and I haven't converted to the eco-friendly car.

As I said, there's a learning curve—of willingness, knowledge, responsibility. As you learn more, you're likely to do more. Just start with one thing, then all of a sudden you're like, *Bamboo floors are awesome! That low-VOC paint comes in such cool colors!* The more I learn, the more these changes make sense. It feels good to make positive changes, ones that improve the health of the people and other living things around me. And I can look my trees in the eye.

Step #3. Paint Without Fumes—and Deal with Lead

Standard household paints release solvents or VOCs. To prevent mold, many paints contain fungicide, too, one of the worst types of pesticide. Oil-based paints are the most overwhelmingly fumey, and should never be used indoors in rooms where kids spend lots of time, but conventional latex, or water-based paints, are also VOC-laden. Even after paint dries, it may still emit an odor, which can worsen when the temperature rises. For most people, it's an annoying stench. For sensitive breathers and asthmatics, it can be an assault on their health.

Fortunately, several big paint companies now make low- and even zero-VOC paint. While these paints may still emit some fumes, they're usually far milder than the standard. (For recommended brands, see

Healthy Resources.) When you paint, keep windows and doors open and use fans to circulate air; when the job's complete, stay out of the room, if possible, for at least a couple days. No matter the paint's VOC content, pregnant women should not wield a brush, however much they're driven by the do-it-before-baby-arrives demon.

Other natural paints, made from citrus, milk protein, or clay are also healthier for you, yours, and the environment because they don't contain preservatives or biocides. They're rich and beautiful—and often quite expensive. Wood stains should be VOC-free, too.

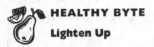 **HEALTHY BYTE**
Lighten Up

If low-VOC paints are too pricey, at least go with a lighter shade of conventional: the darker the paint, the greater the VOC concentration.

Other wall coverings. To prettify your walls with something other than paint, eco-conscientious home improvement stores carry lots of nontoxic finishes and wall coverings, including lime wash/clay finishes, recycled glass tiles, natural stucco (lime and sand combined), cork paper (thin rolls of cork, or cork square tiles for acoustic dampening), ceramic and stone tiles, and natural fiber coverings such as arrowroot, bamboo, cattail, jute, paper weaves, reed, rush, sea grass, or sisal (these may not be ideal in extremely moist rooms). Some manufacturers are producing finished wallboards in place of traditional drywall. For a range of options, see the Healthy Resources section.

Many wallpapers, and certainly the most affordable kinds, are made from vinyl, which releases unhealthy chemicals—as do the chemically potent adhesives used to glue them up. Seek out non-vinyl paper, organic cotton, or recycled content wallpaper, and use a nontoxic paste or adhesive.

Get the lead out. Paint in older homes may contain lead, and in fact, house paint is the number one source of childhood lead poisoning.

Take extreme precaution when sanding or demolishing (and absolutely do not participate if you're pregnant): Even when buried under layers of newer paint, the old layers may generate lead dust, which can contaminate indoor air or the soil around the home. Dr. Philip Landrigan, director of the Center for Children's Health and the Environment at the Mount Sinai School of Medicine, says that approximately 15 percent of the lead poisoning cases he sees in New York are the result of home repair or renovation. If your home was built prior to 1978, or your paint is chipping or deteriorating, then test for lead *before* painting or renovating. If you suspect you have a lead problem, consider hiring a certified lead inspector to evaluate your home; the test kits from hardware stores are far from conclusive, since they can't detect lead below the surface paint. (The December 2007 *Consumer Reports* rated Homax Lead Check, Lead Check Household Lead Test Kit, and Lead Inspector—all under twenty dollars—as the best.) A pro, meanwhile, uses a scanner to see what lies beneath the paint. To find a certified lead testing and removal service (known as "lead abatement"), contact the EPA's National Lead Information Center (epa.gov/oppt/lead/pubs/nlic.htm and click on "Where You Live" for regional offices that can help you; 800-424-LEAD). You can also order their fact sheet, "Reducing Lead Hazards When Remodeling Your Home."

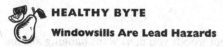 **HEALTHY BYTE**
Windowsills Are Lead Hazards

Lead paint on the inside surfaces of window tracks and the surrounding molding inevitably peels fastest due to vibration, rubbing, and exposure to outdoor weather. Think about where in your home you might be most likely to find paint chips: in window wells. It follows that windowsills are a primary source of lead exposure. Children like to spend time in front of windows, looking outside and even playing with items (like toy cars) that can fit within the window tracks. They have ample opportunity to pick up lead chips and dust on their hands and ingest it from routine hand-to-mouth contact. Perhaps even more dangerous, the paint chips that fall in window wells get ground into a dust that can blow into the house. Therefore, it is especially important to address lead paint in these areas of your house.

Source: **What's Toxic, What's Not** *by Dr. Gary Ginsberg and Brain Toal,* **M.S.P.H.**

Step #4. Armchair (and Other Furniture) Activism

When you bring furniture into your home, be it a foam-filled couch or recently varnished table, it's not just a passive item. If the piece was conventionally made or finished, chances are it's releasing VOCs and other unhealthy fumes into the air. We don't think of furniture as contributing to indoor air pollution, but it's an important factor in the air quality of our homes.

Greening your furniture means introducing pieces that are sustainably produced or from recycled materials that require less energy and resources to make, and reducing their toxic chemical content. In recent years there has been an explosion in modern eco-furniture design, a lot of which looks nothing like the funky blobjects of hippie days. These pieces, often handmade and one of a kind, can strain a budget, but greening your house isn't meant to be an overnight process. Besides, there are plenty of other cost-effective ways to ensure the furniture you keep is healthier for your family.

Good woods. First, a word about woods you *don't* want hanging around your home. So much of our affordable furniture, from shelving to cabinetry, is made from "manufactured" woods—pressed wood and plywood (recognizable by their layer-cake cross-section), and particleboard and chipboard (which looks like wood chips stuck in a cake). These contain glues that give off formaldehyde, a probable carcinogen. However, if you've had a piece in your home for a while, it's probably okay, since it has already given off most of its toxic payload. If you're buying new, consider these greener options:

Independently certified wood furniture. Furnishings certified as sustainable by the Forest Stewardship Council (FSC) contribute less to deforestation, which causes greenhouse gas emissions and messes with natural habitats. Mainstream chain stores and home improvement centers are selling more FSC products each year, so the price is more competitive with regular lumber.

Reclaimed wood. Many people construct pieces out of wood from old furniture, torn-down homes, or factory scraps. Some reclaimed wood even comes from the bottom of rivers where logs sank during transport. Look for the Rainforest Alliance Rediscovered Wood Certification seal.

Unfinished wood furniture. Some furniture and cabinet makers will sell you an unfinished piece, which you can cover, if you choose, with low-VOC, water-based polyurethane stains and sealants, or safe plant oils such as minerals, tung oil, or beeswax.

Seal the deal yourself. With manufactured plywood or particleboard furniture, you can paint a nontoxic sealant on the exposed end of pressed wood to keep toxic chemicals from being released. Do this outdoors or in a well-ventilated room with a mask.

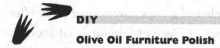

DIY
Olive Oil Furniture Polish

If you've ditched your conventional polish (furniture oil is highly poisonous if ingested), you can buff your wood with natural oils. This is best used on furniture with an oily, rather than glossy, finish. But first test a small section, since using this polish on fine antiques may leave a cloudy haze.

Combine two cups olive oil and one juiced lemon in a glass or ceramic container. Apply to furniture with a soft polishing cloth; rub briskly to shine. Allow furniture to dry. Admire self in reflection.

Re-up your re-upholstery. Most conventional furniture is composed of foam core stuffing, which is treated with flame retardants. If buying

new or getting furniture reupholstered, seek natural foam rubber, organic cotton, and wool fill (or some combo) for the core. As for fabric,
look for types made from organic cotton or silk, which are untreated
and contain low-impact dyes. The cost can be high, but generally in line
with that for comparable high-end furniture, and the materials are incredibly durable.

Avoid hunks of plastic junk. It's almost impossible in this age of conve-
nient, cheap consumption to avoid having plastic around the house; I'm
not advocating a no-tolerance policy. But if you're shopping for, say, a
shelving unit, indoor trash can, or table-and-chair set for the kids, try to
steer clear of those ubiquitous colorful plastics.

Look into other eco-friendly materials. Bamboo isn't a tree but a grass,
and is incredibly fast-growing and versatile. It can be used for flooring,
furniture, window blinds, even fabric. Other green options include recycled plastic and metal, which don't tax the earth's resources as much.
However, keep in mind that plastic *is* plastic.

Give a green thumbs up. A number of groups have sprung up to offer
certification for indoor furnishings. A piece of furniture that sports a
Green Seal adheres to high environmental standards. The Green Seal
report (greenseal.org) on wood finishes lists VOC emissions and chemical ingredient information that might not be obvious from manufacturer
labels. GREENGUARD certification (greenguard.org) also ensures that
furniture is lower in toxicity. And products stamped by McDonough
Braungart Design Chemistry's Cradle to Cradle product standards
(mbdc.com) promote easy repair, disassembly, and recycling at the end
of their life span.

Embrace grandma's attic. When you need stuff, bringing in used
pieces is about the greenest thing you can do for your décor. Pre-
owned, conventionally made furniture has likely already finished off-
gassing, so it won't introduce bad air into your home. Just make sure

old upholstered furniture is in good condition—i.e., no foam core bursting through the cushions, and upholstery that's mold- and dander-free. Say yes to offers from family for old bureaus and desks; haunt local tag sales and flea markets; troll eBay, craigslist, and Freecycle.

Note that old painted wood may contain lead and should not be handled by kids, especially if it's chipped.

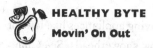

HEALTHY BYTE
Movin' On Out

If your reno project means potentially exposing your family to toxic chemicals—from fumes in paint and carpet to lead, mold, or asbestos—move in with the grandparents or find another place to crash before it all starts, and return only after floor surfaces are clean and the rooms aired out for at least seventy-two hours. That goes double for pregnant women.

Step #5. Make the Lav More Livable

The bathroom is one of the worst-ventilated spaces in the home, so pay attention to air quality in there. And I don't mean by striking a match.

It's curtains. Instead of a conventional vinyl curtain, which releases irritating and harmful fumes, opt for organic cotton, linen, canvas, or hemp, all of which are washable and reusable; and bath mats made of organic cotton or a combo of cotton and bamboo, rather than the rubber-backed kind.

Towel off. For towels and washcloths, look for pesticide-free organic cotton or bamboo, with no trace of triclosan, an antibacterial chemical. You can also find wood fiber towels made with wood pulp. If you're buying regular (nonorganic) towels, wash them first in hot water to remove any unwanted residues.

Ventilate well. Tile and toilet cleansers are among the harshest products made, and fumes can build up in a small space—another reason to use one of the many safer, green cleaners on the market. And because it's the most humid room in the house, bathrooms are petri dishes for mold and mildew. Use your exhaust fan to remove humidity and chemical buildup. If you don't have a fan, investigate having one put in. Note that fans need to exhaust to the outside, and not just recirculate the indoor air.

Down the drain. Consider installing water-saving appliances like low- or dual-flush toilets, faucet aerators, and low-flow showerheads. See Chapter 7 for more information on conserving (and filtering) water.

      # Parentblog

Waiting to Inhale

By Zem Joaquin, founder of ecofabulous.com

One day, conventional cleaning product in hand, I began to have chest pains. Feeling short of breath, my gaze drifted to the product's label (which will remain nameless but feel free to insert your favorite chemical cleaner), and the link suddenly occurred to me: My household products could affect my personal health. As a mother of two children with asthma, I couldn't ignore the larger implication. I was shocked it took me so long to realize. I thought I was doing a healthy thing by removing grime, but in the process I was poisoning myself in some way or, at the very least, experiencing a severe chemical sensitivity. Before that point, I hadn't made the connection between the smells coming from my cleaning products and what was going on in my own home.

Here's what was going on: My children, Dylan and Zoe, had both developed asthma, starting when each was about one. Anytime they got a cold or flu or any type of illness, it inevitably made it into their lungs and they'd wind up having an attack. Every two to three weeks, one of them, sometimes both, would be on a nebulizer; often it got so bad we had to rush them to the ER. To top it off, *I* was getting sick frequently. It seemed I always had bronchitis or some other respiratory problem.

The doctors' solution? Steroids as preventative medicine for the kids, and inhalers always at the ready. But neither of these seemed like sustainable options. Chemical dependency was not something I wished for my children. And always treating them with inhalers didn't eliminate the root cause of their problem; it just managed the symptom.

I realized I'd been exposing my children—and my husband and myself—to all these toxic chemicals in our cleaning products, and in many materials in our home. My life's mission came to me with unbelievable clarity. It's amazing how everything can change in a single moment.

My approach was holistic and thorough. I looked at every material in our house. I'm not going to lie to you: The changes weren't (always) cheap, and it took time and research. But I switched to nontoxic cleaning supplies, to organic mattresses, bedding, and towels; I removed carpets; I put in air and water filters. Was I obsessed? Yes—and I still am. Has our investment paid off? Let's just say that my kids, who recently started a new school year, just came down with colds for the first time this year—astonishing in and of itself. In the past, it always turned into asthma after a couple of days; not this time. Actually, they haven't had a single incident in over a year and a half! And I've never felt better.

Step #6. Appliance Yourself

Most of the health issues surrounding appliances and electronics have more to do with the world outside your home (conserving energy and water, reducing pollution, keeping plastic and metals out of landfills) than the one inside (eliminating exposure). When you're ready to replace an appliance, it makes sense to buy a piece of equipment that's Energy Star–rated for its superior efficiency: It consumes less energy, which helps both the environment and your finances. But there are a few points to consider about appliances, electronics, and your family's health.

A cleaner cooker. When buying a gas stove, consider one with an electronic ignition rather than a pilot light. It's not only more efficient but it eliminates the continuous low-level gas pollutants that can emanate from the pilot light, which can contribute to breathing difficulties and irritate asthmatics. (If the flame's color has excessive yellow in it, call your appliance repair service—yellow means the pilot light isn't burning clean.) Install an effective outside-exhausting ventilation hood—and use it regularly—to reduce these levels.

Washer woes. When they're working, top-loading clotheswashers and most dishwashers put quite a bit of soapy, chemical-laden humidity into your home's air. For this reason, front-loading washers are better; they're sealed during operation. Or install an outside-exhausting vent fan in your laundry room and make sure it runs during the wash cycle.

Dryer idea. Make sure the dryer exhaust vent is clean so that particles don't ventilate back into the house. Of course, a clothesline is the greenest way to dry laundry.

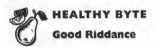 **HEALTHY BYTE**
Good Riddance

If you're doing a reno and want to keep your old appliance out of the landfill, consult with Earth 911 (earth911.org), the source for information on recycling and disposing of everything in your home in a safer, healthier way.

Earth-friendlier electronics. All electronics contain toxic chemicals and heavy metals—flame retardants, lead, cadmium, and mercury, to name a few. While exposure isn't a likely problem for casual users, some elevated levels of flame retardants have shown up in the blood of superfrequent users. There's not much one can do about this; it's where computers (and TVs and stereos and other electronic appliances) end up that carries bigger health consequences.

Electronics are the number one source of individual hazardous waste. By recycling old electronics, you keep chemicals out of the ecosystem—and ultimately our water and air. A few other green schemes: Sell your outdated gadgetry online; there are people out there who buy them even when broken. Also, more computer manufacturers are instituting take-back programs, and will accept and recycle their own units. Alternatively, donate your computer to a local school or look into the Computers for Schools program (pcsforschools.org). For more recycling and donation ideas, see the Healthy Resources section.

70

percentage of all hazardous waste that comes from electronics.

(worldchanging.com, 2005)

Fortunately, some electronics may now be a bit lighter on harmful substances, thanks to Europe's launch of the Restriction on Hazardous Substances (RoHS) initiative, which limits levels of some toxic pollutants. To find products that meet RoHS standards, visit greenelectronics .com, greenercomputing.com, or mygreenelectronics.org. More help: the EPA's Electronic Product Environmental Assessment Tool (EPEAT). It evaluates models by fifty-one environmental criteria, including chemicals and recyclable parts (epeat.net).

Step #7. Insulation Solutions

Conventional fiberglass insulation, which accounts for 90 percent of all residential insulation sold and installed in the United States, is made from silica spun into glass fiber. Traditionally it has contained formaldehyde, though formaldehyde-free fiberglass insulation is getting easier to find. Either way, though, when fiberglass is cut or damaged, tiny microscopic shards of glass go airborne, sometimes settling in the lungs.

Green's getting good props here, too: Various healthier products have hit the market, some cellulose-based (made from postconsumer recycled cardboard), others bio-based or made of soybean. Some are spray-in and some go in dry. One material gaining in popularity is recycled and reclaimed denim (cotton). These alternative insulators are free of chemical additives and flame retardants.

What's best for you depends on the climate, particularly humidity. Before installing insulation, seek credible professional advice; one man's straw bale insulation is another man's moldy pile of muck.

Parentblog
Body (Burden) of Evidence
By Laura Turner Seydel, chair of Captain Planet Foundation, builder of ecomanor.com.

My father, my son, and I all had our "body burden" assessed by the Environmental Working Group. It was the first study on the impact of environmental toxins across three generations. Our blood and urine were tested for eighty-four chemicals in ten chemical groups. My sample contained thirty-nine of the eighty-four. All three of us showed evidence of plasticizers, Teflon, flame retardants, lead, and mercury (to name just a few). Not surprisingly, of the three of us, I showed the highest levels of musks, which are fragrance chemicals in cosmetics, detergents, and air fresheners. I also showed the highest levels of phthalates, a plasticizer found in PVC food containers, vinyl flooring, and personal care products. But what really concerned me was that my son showed the greatest level of chemicals overall, as well as the highest exposure of perchlorate, an ingredient in rocket fuel that contaminates the food supply, including produce and dairy. He also topped us on various flame retardants—an unexpected finding since they tend to accumulate over years. Could it be that his level was so high (and perhaps mine, which was lower than his but higher than my dad's) because they're found in TVs and computers? (They're also in furniture and carpet padding.) Of course we all had mercury. That's pretty worrisome. These body burden tests are a good wake-up call for why it's important to eat healthy, to stay away from mercury-heavy big-game fish, to limit your exposure to things like popcorn microwaved in Teflon-lined bags, and even bottled water. Although I knew of tests that revealed all these toxic chemicals in people's bodies—even in newborns'—it's sobering to find out what's actually in your own.

Step #8. Blowing Hot and Cold

Your home's capacity to regulate temperature goes a long way in determining its comfort. Improving how well your home cools and heats through passive strategies or vents, fans, and air-conditioning lessens the strain on the systems and can also improve air quality.

Be passive aggressive. South-facing windows can be agents of temperature control. Either let them heat up a room, greenhouse-style, or cover them with solar shades, which block sunlight and heat. You can find show-off quality shades in green materials including grasses, reeds, bamboo, and hemp. Drapes, too, come in 100 percent organic cotton and silk.

Of course, windows themselves go a long way toward determining energy efficiency. On a windy day, hold a lighter or candle and go around the perimeter of a window; if the flame flickers or goes out, you've got a draft. Caulking, weather-stripping, or installing energy-efficient windows will make your home less drafty and lower your heating bills.

Update your HVAC (heating, ventilation, and air-conditioning system). Your house's network of ducts is part of your HVAC; leaky ducts not only rob your air conditioner or heating system's performance but also affect indoor air quality. It's not unusual for a home duct system to leak 25 percent or more of its air during operation, creating negative air pressure, which in turn causes the house to suck in more mold, pollens, and pollutants from those dark, damp places—such as the crawl space under the house, attic, or attached garage.

Your biggest fan. With a good ceiling fan installed, you can raise your air conditioner setting by several degrees—and improve respiratory health.

It's okay to say it: *I own, use, and love my air conditioner.* If you rely on one—and those prone to asthma and other respiratory issues will

benefit from air-conditioning on hot and muggy or high pollution index days—then at least make sure it's the right size for your needs.
Oversized air-conditioning systems never run during their typical cycle
for a long enough period to really dehumidify or filter your air effectively.

Furthermore, if you've first followed all the passive cooling strategies
and made energy-saving improvements, then you won't have to use your
air-conditioning unit quite so much. When you do turn it on, you can
probably keep it at a temperature a couple degrees higher than you're
used to without feeling a difference.

BURNING QUESTION
What's up with electromagnetic fields?

Electromagnetic fields (EMFs) are fields created by energy use around
the home, emitted by outlets, appliances, and electronic chargers. There
are no definitive studies on the effects of EMFs on health, though there
is evidence that excessive exposure to magnetic fields is associated with
an elevation in childhood leukemia. It's worth taking precautions to
minimize EMFs, so keep your child at least four feet from TV sets. A
CD player with white noise is great for helping babies sleep but plug it
in at least a few feet from the crib. If you use an electric blanket, heat
it before getting in bed, then turn it off. If you're concerned about
EMFs, buy a gaussmeter from a home improvement store and periodically test your outlets and appliances to measure the level of emissions.

For more information, see The Bioinitiative Report (bioinitiative.org).
This report also deals with radio-frequency radiation, as from cell phones,
and offers suggestive evidence that kids who use cell phones excessively
court a higher risk of brain cancer.

Step #9. Bright Lights, Big Smile

Studies show that natural sunlight beamed indoors—in homes, offices,
and schools—makes us happier, more productive, and maybe even more

resistant to getting sick; Seasonal Affective Disorder (SAD), in which sufferers feel melancholy, slumpy, and sleep-deprived, strikes a half million adults in the United States. The more natural light you can get, the better. It also means less burning of fossil fuels.

Keep on the sunny side. If you're renovating, add skylights or south-facing windows for maximum exposure. If you don't have room for a full skylight, try solar tubes (available at home improvement stores), which are inserted in the ceiling/roof and funnel narrow beams of natural light into the room below.

Brighten after dark. Look for high-quality fluorescents, including compact fluorescent lightbulbs (CFLs)—those corkscrew-like tubes that wallop incandescent bulbs on the efficiency front. Once a novelty, CFLs take less than a minute (no lightbulb jokes) to swap in. True, CFL light can be harsh, but many of the newest fluorescents give off a warmer glow. When buying a CFL, look for its color temperature, measured in Kelvins (K); a range between 2650 and 3000K yields pretty warm light. A CFL costs more upfront but because it lasts so much longer and costs so much less to operate than an incandescent, you'll save money, energy, and hassle (instead of changing the bulb once a year, say, it's more like once every *seven*). Note: Even CFLs contain mercury, and should be recycled rather than tossed in the trash.

Other ways to save on light energy consumption:

Darken empty rooms. A lighting rule of thumb, for when you exit the room: Shut off incandescents if you'll be gone even for just seconds; for CFLs, kill them if you're away more than three minutes; for standard fluorescents, more than fifteen minutes.

Add dimmers, motion sensors and/or timers (though CFLs have to be rated for dimming).

Step #10. Renovate Intelligently

If you're planning a much more extensive job—a renovation or complete gut—then you can make ground-level choices that are healthy all the way around—physically, environmentally, financially. Here are a few goals that experienced green builders encourage:

Do not disturb. A couple of chemicals found in older homes can be hazardous if released. Asbestos can still be found in some houses in insulation around pipes and furnaces and on walls and ceilings (especially as sprayed-on material) and drop-ceiling panels. The danger is that, when disturbed, asbestos can be released as a fine dust and eventually get caught in lungs (in extreme cases, as with workers who handled the material, causing cancer—though the risk of this is very low for residential exposure). If you plan to tear down walls or redo an attic and your home was built before 1973 and contains any of the aforementioned suspect tiles or insulation, hire a professional asbestos manager to test your home and remove any asbestos found. State and local health departments can refer you to approved labs, or log on to epa.gov/asbestos/pubs/regioncontact.html.

Lead in paint is generally safe if it remains covered (though you have to stay on top of cracks and peeling areas); however, the chance of exposure increases very significantly during a renovation when walls are taken down and/or sanded. See Step #3 for more info.

Clean your mess without making a new one. A three-hundred-square-foot kitchen remodel generates about twenty-eight cubic yards of debris. Yet it's only fairly recently that builders have seriously tried to recycle such waste. Make sure your contractor understands the benefits of "deconstruction" over demolition: It conserves natural resources and reduces pressure on landfills. Set aside space to separate materials for reuse, including lumber, hardware, tile, water heaters, molding, windows, doors, sinks and tubs, bricks, and appliances. Salvage, reuse, donate, or sell everything possible. Post big items like stoves and refrigerators on freecycle.org or donate them to charities such as Habitat for Humanity (habitat.org). Plus, you reduce disposal costs.

Work with what you have. As best you can, exploit your natural, topographical surroundings: sunlight for day lighting and heating purposes, wind for cross-ventilation. And while tearing down an existing structure and replacing it and most of its contents—even for something "green"—may sound like homeowner nirvana, in fact it runs counter to the very nature of sustainability. If you can green what's already there, it will be far less wasteful.

Think long-term. For all the cost of green improvements, upgrading smartly yields significant savings, year after year, more than making up for the often higher upfront expense.

 ONE STEP BEYOND

Do a home energy audit. This is especially important if you're about to buy a new system (air conditioner, windows, solar water heater, etc.). You can conduct the audit yourself by doing a walk-through of your home, making a list of obvious drafts, checking for gaps along the baseboard or junctures where wall meets floor or ceiling, and fixing accordingly. (See the U.S. Department of Energy's Do It Yourself Home Energy Audits guide at eere.energy.gov/consumer/your_home/energy_audits and click on "Do It Yourself.") Or have a licensed professional make a thorough evaluation: They should do a room-by-room inspection, run tests, and examine your past utility bills. Afterward they'll offer advice on everything from tree shading/removal to air-conditioning systems, which can translate to significant energy and financial savings.

Generate your own. The most common way to brew your own energy juice is to install photovoltaic (PV) panels. These "solar panels," mounted on rooftops or the ground, harness the sun's energy, and convert it to electricity. The system is an initial investment upfront but pays for itself over time and you'll notice clear cost savings right away on your electric bill. Since building codes are constantly changing to incorporate new technologies, check yours before investing in a solar solution.

❧ Expert Opinion ❧
Remaking Our Design
By William McDonough, architect, designer, coauthor of
Cradle to Cradle: Remaking the Way We Make Things

From 1994 until 1999, my family and I had the privilege of living at the University of Virginia in a house designed by Thomas Jefferson. We celebrated the astonishing architecture and landscape legacies that he created, and I came to appreciate that Mr. Jefferson saw himself, first and last, as a designer: One of his final creations—his tombstone—records only the things he made. *Thomas Jefferson*, it reads. *Author of the Declaration of American Independence, of the Statute of Virginia for Religious Freedom and Father of The University of Virginia.* That's it. No mention of his having been President of the United States, or Minister to France, or all the other things he did. He chose to record his legacies, not his activities.

Design is the first signal of human intention. The legacies Jefferson left are extraordinary because—consummate designer that he was—he had the best of intentions. What will future generations make of our design—this modern industrialized world, and our way of making and using things? If we perpetuate this way, across many enterprises, then it seems as if our legacy will be tragic, *intentionally* so, marked by climate change, endocrine disruption, persistent toxification, plastic pollution in the oceans, and dramatic loss of species diversity. We as a species have released thousands of chemicals into the environment, many of which harm our children and the children of other species. While certainly that was never our intention, how will future generations ever know that, given the legacy we leave?

It's time to question our design. As the dominant species, the epic choices before us, especially now, are marked by dramatically different intentions, which lead to dramatically different legacies. The new design must be full of hope. Our design assignment at this moment in our history could, perhaps, be summed up thus: Make a world where we love all the children of all species for all time. If that were the plan, then we'd have no choice but to create a world that is safe, healthy, and just, with clean air, water, soil, and power; a world that is delightfully diverse, economically equitable, ecologically sound, elegant, and enjoyable.

How might we create such a paradise? For a practical species such as ours, we'd have to imagine all the many steps that would go into making this ideal state. In our firm, we are inspired by what we call "cradle to cradle" thinking, which is premised on respect for each component of the design: the large-scale system one is making—the end product—as well as all the parts that make it up, and the material that makes up those parts. In this new design of ours, we would be obligated to evince concern for the Earth as well as all the organisms on it, as well as the very molecules that make up everything. For example, we would fully appreciate the large-scale system that has provided almost all energy through history—the sun—as well as the smallest components our planet is blessed with—such as the tiny, intensely valuable hydrocarbons that make up fossil fuels. Lately, though, we have not shown appropriate concern for these component parts, which have an almost infinite number of uses when made into polymers and other objects of human need and desire. If we properly valued them, then why on earth would we burn them, turning them into a liability for the planet? Yet we have right now between five and ten thousand times the energy we need to operate every day, if we could only commit fully to developing renewable energy sources such as wind and solar power.

There's another profound casualty to our current faulty design, perhaps just as toxic as what we do: how we think. Because of the fear of depleted resources, many people have developed a mentality characterized by limitation. *How much can I get?* they wonder. *How little can I give?* That way of thinking is just as much a part of our design, too.

There's no reason to perpetuate this current bad design, no reason for us to continue to use materials that are toxic to our species, no reason we can't put what we know about clean production to good effect. But we must respect equally the whole and the parts of the system, or the design must falter. In a cradle-to-cradle world, we don't produce hazardous products or waste. In fact, we eliminate the concept of waste. One entity's waste is another one's food. All goods become good.

The impact of this new design strategy? Abundance. Millions of new jobs (in renewable energy and elsewhere). Access for many more people to clean air, water, soil, and power.

And this abundance also means, not insignificantly, a new way of thinking. *How much can I get?* will become *How much can I give?* We can achieve that.

CHAPTER 10

It's All Good

HOW TO GROW YOUR IMPACT

I f you've gotten this far, then presumably you've taken some action in your home—tossing out conventional cleaning products, for instance, or reading labels more diligently, or swapping plastic drinking bottles for stainless steel. Maybe you've done all that and more. You deserve huge praise for anything you did.

More can be done, too. While we first want to address the environment's effect on our kids, we should also consider *our* impact on the surroundings. That means taking action outside the home. What's your passion—promoting awareness of food allergies? Reducing pesticides in your neighborhood? Ridding your daughter's school of unhealthy cleaning products? Can you figure out how realistically to have the greatest impact on that issue? While it may sound Pollyannaish to insist that every voice counts, as you'll see in the points to follow, every voice *does* count; too many instances bear this out. In the words of The Body Shop founder Anita Roddick, "If you think you're too small to have an impact, try going to bed with a mosquito."

Step #1. Get Smart

You're spooked, engaged, hopeful, enraged, fired up. Stuff needs to be done in your home, your life, the world . . . but where to start? To determine which actions or lifestyle modifications will yield the best buck-bang, first understand your *own* situation better.

Educate yourself. Spend a night Googling a subject—ingredients in your cosmetics, your county's pesticide policy, ways to test your water, whatever. Terrific resources are posted by government agencies, watchdog and advocacy groups, university departments, and education-oriented green sites. (Or start with some of the names in our Healthy Resources section.) Once you start, chances are you'll be hooked.

Go through what's already in your home. Contemplate what you regularly bring into it. Assess the issues plaguing (or not plaguing) *your* water and air, your diet, your garden, etc.; understand how the choices you've made about your home affect your health. (Does your basement playroom—a poorly ventilated space where your children come and play with their toys—have conventional wall-to-wall carpeting? Why? Would it be worth rethinking flooring options?)

Read labels: on food, cleaning, and personal care products, and any other purchases you make for your household. Keep a log for one week, documenting what you buy, discard, use most, or not at all. One, this allows you to assess your home's actual needs and, two, it's empowering. You're taking control of your lifestyle.

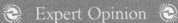

✺ Expert Opinion ✺
Dig, Trust, Fight . . . and Fight Some More
By Erin Brockovich, environmental activist, Healthy Child
Healthy World board member

To bring about change, the most important thing is information. If the issue is pesticides, then find out and isolate who in your area is using them and for what purpose. If it's on a large enough scale to affect the community, are there airplanes spraying overhead? Pick up a phone. The Freedom of Information Act gives you access to records. Go to your county department of records, find out who's doing it, what they're using, what its effects are. Lots of times there's a Material Safety Data Sheet (MSDS). I know it sounds like a lot, but there's always one angry mom in the group who's willing to do the research. It doesn't matter if you're dealing with public agencies, Congress, neighbors: If you go into a tirade without facts, it will fall on deaf ears. (If you don't like to speak publicly, work with someone who can; none of us is ever a lone warrior.) But when you have documents, when you can say, *This is poison being sprayed. . . . Look at how often they're spraying. . . .* People are masters at making connections. *Oh, my god, my daughter has been acting like that, too.* As soon as it hits home, as soon as it's about parent and child and neighborhood, people spring into action.

First, though, you need to make the connection. I'm an advocate for common sense. If an exterminator uses a chemical that makes a spider drop dead right in front of you, what's its effect on a child? Ask questions. Don't be afraid to say, *I don't want you to do that.* As the mom, the one who knows her children better than anyone, rely on your gut instinct. I'll argue with doctors if they say something I know is not true about my child. When you have questions, I believe it's your human barometer working for you. I frequently lecture about how social intimidation and peer pressure can take away our common sense, make us back away from gut feelings. It happened to me. They said, *What do you know about science? You don't have a Ph.D., you're not a lawyer, why should we listen to you?* Why? Because there's a lot that I *do* know, that we all know. I was born in Kansas and when I see a tornado, I don't need to call an expert to know I should run. When I see a poison, when I know what I'm feeling and seeing, don't tell me otherwise.

You need stick-to-it-iveness. I did two seasons of a television series focusing on women who never stopped or gave up on their cause. The things you think will get results and work out, won't; so you have to keep coming back and coming back. They say you catch more flies with honey but the squeaky wheel gets the grease.

And then you have to listen to people—honestly, without preconceptions. One mistake I made that I vowed never to do again: Do not disregard what anyone says to you, even if it sounds ludicrous. When you think you know everything, you don't open yourself up. People told me bizarre things that happened to them and their animals when they were exposed, and I didn't believe them at first. I would think, *Are you on acid?* They would tell me they had cancer and I was thinking, *How can you have cancer when you look so well?* No, that can't happen, that doesn't happen. Only it turns out that it can, and it does. So don't be deceived because you can't see something. No one knows you but you. A child can be stung by a bee a hundred times and it doesn't bother him, and the next time it does; or another kid is affected on the very first sting. Everyone is different. Don't ever get too certain about what you think is true.

Step #2. Pass It On

Neighbors, friends, local merchants: There are others like you out there, with similar fears, hopes, and exposure to risk, only they may be unaware of those risks or what can be done about them. Spread your newfound knowledge. They benefit and so do you, by helping your community raise accountability. Here are some simple ways to let others know what you know:

Say it in a community newsletter. Ask to write a blurb about children's health and environmental impacts; whatever size the paper's subscriber base, it's usually a committed readership.

Do something special on PTA night/bake sale day/school open house. Ask to set up a table with fact sheets about children's health and the environment. Probably they'll say yes (so long as the venue is appropriate) since parents who volunteer or hold school leadership positions are typically civic-minded.

Or start a green committee at your child's school. Recruiting parents won't be hard since most of them are thinking about issues like improving school lunches, the availability of snack and soda vending machines, recycling, beautifying school grounds with plantings, finding a way to add outdoor or gym time, bringing in naturalists to teach kids about worms and composting—you name it.

Go online. Countless virtual communities share information, ask and answer questions, and just schmooze about a better way. Join one and spread the word—though try not to preach, or you risk turning off those otherwise eager to listen. Blog. Comment on posts or items you see online.

Find others like you. "Think global, act local," they say, but you can think and act in both ways at once. At earthshare.org, click on "Get Involved" and link to a host of well-respected, big-picture organizations engaged in environmental efforts—National Audubon Society, The Nature Conservancy, Sierra Club, Rails-to-Trails Conservancy, and the National Parks Conservation Association. Select the local/regional chapter or your state, and find a calendar of events, where to volunteer, and learn more. See volunteermatch.org for other national and international opportunities. Numerous areas on meetup.com are devoted to activism.

 HEALTHY BYTE
Write a Letter to the Editor (That Actually Gets Published)

Your neighbors read the letters section in the local paper, so getting your ideas out there about environmental health can whip up local interest. To increase your chance of getting published, here are some guidelines:

- Outline the problem, support with facts, spell out a solution. Describe what individuals and organizations are doing in your area, and how to get involved.

- **The more personal, the better. The briefer, the better.**
- **Refer to a recent story.** An article about health, education, or the environment can serve as your "hook."
- **Tap into national issues but give them local spin.** Newspaper people are wired into the big stories; tell how your community is affected.
- **Submit underexposed topics.** Editorial pages need a mix.
- **Link to multimedia.** If possible, submit with photos, links, and video clips. It's no guarantee they'll be included, but you probably better your chance by providing more than just text.
- **Build relationships.** Opinion page departments tend to have little turnover. Work with them, provide credible facts, and be open to edits.
- **Identify to whom and where to send your letter.** The editor's name should be at the top of the op-ed page. Call the department for any info you need to know to be taken seriously. Ask for word count limit. Submit it via regular mail or electronically.
- **Forget your Pulitzer-winning headline.** The op-ed staff crafts it.

Finally, if you're writing to more than one paper—a good idea—know that each letter should be unique. Papers don't (knowingly) publish letters printed elsewhere.

Step #3. Play Detective

Examine the public environments your kids frequent. Walk through their school or child-care facility, alert to potential exposure risks. Talk with teachers and child-care providers, respectfully, about environmental hazards you've learned about—exposures that can have an impact on kids' health and development, especially when the exposure is daily, as it is at school or day care, for anywhere from two to ten hours—and the simple remedies to follow. While they're likely doing their best to safeguard your kids, they may be unaware of hidden dangers; unsafe cleaning products are typically the biggest culprits. *Creating Healthy Environments for Children*, a DVD created by Healthy Child, offers easy ways for teachers and day-care personnel to learn and take action; go to healthychild.org to find out more.

You can lead the way to minor but meaningful improvements by initiating a (nonconfrontational) conversation with a few basic questions:

Do the windows open? Opening windows for even a few minutes a day, especially in a stuffy, crowded classroom, can significantly improve indoor air quality (though one also needs to beware of outdoor air quality alerts for ozone or allergens). Ask about the HVAC system and the kind of air filters used.

Do trucks, buses, and cars load or idle near the building? Children (adults, too) should not be exposed to vehicle exhaust, especially diesel. Loading or idling areas should be as far as possible from outdoor air intakes and windows. Speak to an administrator about promoting a "No Idling" policy. (Learn more at epa.gov/cleanschoolbus.)

Are renovations and repairs completed? Renovations mean dust and an array of products that release chemicals into the air. Is the school scheduling the work for vacation break or summer? Child-care facilities pose more of a challenge. Ask someone if there's a plan to control dust, fumes, and noise.

Do they use the least toxic cleaning supplies? The stuff schools use can be even more caustic than the conventional ones used in homes. Fortunately, green institutional-grade cleaning products are widely available and cost-effective. See greencleanschools.org for an easy guide and list of available products.

Are the art supplies free of toxic substances? Some classroom supplies, such as markers, glues, and craft materials, contain asbestos, formaldehyde, or solvents. See Chapter 5 for safer alternatives.

Does the school control pests and unwanted weeds without pesticides? If pesticides are used, ask when, where, and for what purpose. Are parents notified prior to pesticide applications? Ask them to consider using Integrated Pest Management (IPM) recommended by the EPA (epa.gov/pesticides/ipm).

 BURNING QUESTION
Seriously now . . . can one person really make a difference?

Almost all our great novels, paintings, inventions, mathematical formulas, business ideas, and jokes came from an individual's vision. Sure, lots of civilization's finest achievements are the result of collaborative effort but history overflows with stories of individuals whose passion and willingness to risk have shaped and improved our world.

Too rah-rah? Still skeptical that one vote can make a difference? Believe it or not, our elected officials generally vote according to how their constituents tell them to. If they get four thousand calls and e-mails in favor of a bill and three thousand against, they vote for it; if it's ten for—not ten thousand, just ten—and twelve against, they vote against it. In Massachusetts, it once took three phone calls to change the whole assembly's opinion about a major children's health bill. It's not rocket science. Representatives simply represent the majority . . . *of those who speak up.*

Step #4. Take the Local

Back in the day, we did it all locally—procured food and gathered building materials from nearby, and built where we stood. Then again, it's not as if we had a choice: The means did not yet exist to easily transport food and lumber. Now? We sit in a restaurant and dine on sea bass from Chile, grapefruits from Florida, Brie from France. Our home might contain furniture made of British Columbia cedar, bamboo flooring from China, or carpet from North Africa.

In many ways, this is a good development—opening markets, creating jobs, bolstering economies, diversifying choices. In other ways, it's bad—fossil fuels are needlessly burned to transport food and materials thousands of miles to places that are already abundant with them; ecosystems are infiltrated by nonindigenous organisms; the disconnect grows between our means and ends, how we live and who makes that happen. Bringing the mountain to Mohammed is impressive, but comes at great cost.

Where you can, buy locally produced food: Support area farms, establish relationships with those who grow the stuff you put in your body (shoppers at farmers' markets, claims one study, converse ten times more than shoppers in supermarkets), and help to reduce the environmental damage caused by transporting your food great distances. Besides knowing more about the food you're eating, you'll probably find it tastier, too. Precisely because it's local, there are no great national directories that list local farms and farmers' markets but just a little searching online should yield a site or organization for virtually any region.

And by buying local—not just food but other goods, too—and by building local, you support businesses with community ties, reduce energy strain, and encourage the replenishment of whatever is consumed. There are great efficiencies to embracing what's right before us, the community in which we live and work, the native geology and topography and crops. After all, they're native to the area for a reason.

Parentblog
New World Options, Old World Values
By Tom Hanks, actor, and Rita Wilson, actress

Tom: Things have changed. Back in the counterculture days, when recycling really started, I did a newspaper drive. Now we all have recycling bins and just do it by habit. My kids grew up recycling. For them, it's ingrained, as normal as putting milk back in the refrigerator.

Rita: Our youngest son is into these shoes made completely from recycled materials. He also wants to change all the lightbulbs in our house to CFLs. But the idea of energy conservation has permeated everyone's consciousness in our family. The kids and I are fanatics about turning off lights. I don't know why I'm like that but we only use a light when we're in that room—working, eating. I try not to have any lights on when people aren't in the room. We also unplug lots of things, like chargers, when they're not in use.

T: We're putting solar panels in the office so that we make electricity and help to power the grid. There's a great program we're involved with now where, for each solar panel you put in your business, BP will put an equal number of solar panels somewhere in a disadvantaged area.

R: Our understanding of energy has changed dramatically. Somehow, when we were younger, we thought it took more energy to turn lights off than to leave them on.

T: Which is false. That's been disproved.

R: Same with cars. We thought you used more gas if you turned it off and on rather than let it idle.

T: Also not true. The story back then was that you wore out the starter. Now it's all electronic ignitions. And if you have an all-electric car, like I do, your mind-set changes in other ways. You never look at a gas station and think about pumping gas. In fact, the only time you might even consider stopping at a gas station is to get a drink or some beef jerky.

R: We've made other changes that seem like a return to the past. For instance, we use no blowers in the yard.

T: It also reduces the noise. The gardener actually uses a rake. Think of that! And we use pesticide *only* when it absolutely has to be used. My brother is an entomologist and he'll suggest to me, Well, if you have *these* pests, then release *those* bugs.

R: We have a clothesline and I still line-dry my sheets. I grew up with no dryer, with our clothes being line-dried. We like it like that. Clothespins and everything.

T: And the sheets smell so much better. If you can't do everything on the line, then at least do the sheets and maybe the bath towels, because they take so much energy to dry.

R: We love simple pleasures. Tom loves anything you wind up.

T: I love wind-up radios. I belong to this organization called the Freeplay Foundation that's giving wind-up radios to orphaned children in Rwanda, so they can have contact with an adult presence, through the radio. You just wind up the radio and, if there's any kind of signal, you get up to a half hour; no external electricity needed. We're also developing a mosquito net with tiny LED lightbulbs. Wind it up and it lights up, no electricity.

R: If I get involved in something or make a change, it's not as if I sit around and say, *Today, I'll make a change*. It's an education process. It's a life-style attitude you develop. Recently I replaced most of our plastic bottles with reusable glass canisters.

T: This new attitude has been developing, I think, since about forty years ago, when Apollo 8 orbited the moon at the end of 1968 and took that first-ever picture of the whole Earth. I remember what an amazing moment that was for everybody, seeing this blue and white ball. *So that's what it looks like*, I thought: *That's all there is*. It felt almost chromosomal: We could see we were limited, that there was not an infinite amount of everything. And that we'd better not waste anything.

Because that's all there was.

Step #5. Re: Re: Re: Everything
(Or As Much As You Can)

We've created more than we need of so many things—a lot more. In many cases, we'll be stuck with them for centuries. So there's huge incentive to "re" everything we can, depending on its function, composition, and condition:

Reduce. In short, use less. In 1960, the average American created 2.7 pounds of waste daily; in 2001, it was 4.4 pounds. Of all the "re"s, reducing is the most important because it's the most effective: It demands no new materials or processes, no cost in new energy. We needn't think up inspired new ways to do something with that which isn't. But reducing means more than, well, reducing: It means also that when we *are* in acquiring mode, we seek durable, long-lasting products and materials—which, over time, will ease our ability to reduce further.

Recycle. Turn a product or material at the end of its usefulness into raw material for another. What percentage of waste do Americans recycle? Most people I ask guess 2 percent, 1 percent, sometimes less. In fact, we recycle about one-third of our waste, double what it was fifteen years ago. If we continue to improve at that rate, how might our environment benefit in the next decade?

Reuse. Fix, donate, trade, or sell an item rather than junking it. From an environmental standpoint, reusing is better even than recycling, because no new processing is required. To make money, use auction sites like ebay.com; to swap or give away items for free, visit freecycle.org, ecyclebin .com, or the many local community portals where you post a message about the item and may well find someone who wants or needs it. (Freecycle boasts participation in seventy-five countries and claims it keeps three hundred tons a day out of landfills.)

Repurpose. Take something whose usefulness (to you) has run out and transform it into something of new utility. This requires more innovation, perhaps, than the other "re"s but may be the most satisfying. Turn shoeboxes into storage containers, an old T-shirt into a cloth grocery bag, old clothes into quilts. Turn almost anything into art, jewelry, coffee tables. When I was a kid, my father took an old door, added legs and clear lacquer (most likely toxic), and suddenly we had a beautiful coffee table; he cut a large wine cask in half . . . voilà, two end tables. Sites like instructables.com, part of the growing DIY movement, provide instructions on repurposing simple household items into stuff like unusually realistic Halloween costumes, musical instruments, and an iPod dock. If you're not handy or inclined yourself, help groups that do this—like kenanausa.com, which supports Kenyan women making wool toys from old scarves and hats.

By following the four Rs, the overall effect on the environment, not to mention our increasingly overcluttered homes, will be rewarding, reha-bilitative, remarkable, resplendent.

HEALTHY BYTE
Representative Democracy Is a Contact Sport

To be one of those voices that speaks up, get in touch with your federal and state elected officials. Go to congress.org and enter your zip code; you'll find names and contact info, access to bills being reviewed, and sign-up for e-mail updates and alerts telling you how your representa-tives vote on each bill. For what's happening with environmental health legislation, state by state, visit the National Conference of State Legisla-tures Web site, ncsl.org, and search "environmental health." To contact local officials, check online for the Web site for your city, county, or school district; while there may not be one dedicated to legislative hap-penings in the community, the Web should yield details about policy news.

When a national vote is pending on a bill you care about:

1. Call your representative's office (within two weeks of the voting).
2. Tell the secretary, "My name is X and I'd like Representative Y to vote for/against Bill ABC." Your call will be recorded. You needn't justify your position. It takes thirty seconds.

Of course, connecting with your representatives is the second step; voting is first. As an election nears, visit Project Vote Smart (vote-smart.org) and enter a candidate's name or your zip code to learn bio-graphical information, voting records, campaign finance sources, and more. They claim they know more about candidates than the candi-dates themselves do.

Step #6. Take It Outside

By now, you know we spend far more time indoors than out, which is
why indoor air quality is such a concern. But the current generation
of keyboard-facile, multimedia-saturated kids spends *far* more time
inside than their parents did, a worrisome jump in just the last decade or so that has been cited as a reason for everything from de-
pression to learning disabilities to diminished physical fitness and
obesity (there are more than three times as many obese children
aged six to eleven today as in 1970). Between 1981 and 1997, the
number of hours that American kids aged six to eight spent playing
outdoors dropped by four per week, while the number of hours in
school went up by five. Bike riding is way down; in the last five years,
scooter riding and skateboarding decreased, too. In roughly the last
decade, the percentage of kids aged seven to eleven who swim, fish,
play touch football, canoe, and water-ski has shrunk by about a
third. And unstructured, unsupervised outdoor time has particularly
bottomed out: While a significant portion of kids do play organized
soccer and baseball, American children spend an average of thirty
minutes of unstructured time outdoors . . . *each week*. In a study of
830 mothers, 70 percent said they played outdoors daily as kids,
compared with 31 percent of their children. Where do the extra
hours go? Kids eight to eighteen spend six-plus hours a day with TV,
electronic games, the computer, and other screens and audio. Many
kids are more engaged by virtual versions of outdoor play—skateboarding and football video games, for example—than the real
thing.

In his book *Last Child in the Woods*, Richard Louv dubs this epidemic "nature deficit disorder." Certainly there are valid cultural and
generational reasons for it: More households with two working parents
or single parents; media-fueled fears of child predators running amok;
greater suburban sprawl; more homework (for America's youngest children, the amount has tripled since 1981); maybe even superior video

game graphics. But the connection that so many children now lack with the outdoors is bound to lead to further disconnection as they grow up—How can they love what they don't really know?—as well as other diminishments. (In one intergenerational study, the number of people who reported that the outdoors was the most influential environment of their childhood dropped from 96 percent to 46 percent.) Aside from the obvious physical benefits of being outside, studies show that more outdoor time equals greater competence in negotiating the larger world, the chance to develop courage, and longer attention span. Breathing fresh *outdoor* air, swimming in a clean lake or ocean, playing ball, just plain running around, gardening, climbing trees, learning the ways of plants and animals, and interacting with others are intrinsically worthwhile activities, plus they cultivate an awareness of, and appreciation for, how our physical environment works, its rhythms, and what's needed to maintain its vitality. After all, this generation of children is the next generation of botanists, zoologists, marine biologists, and naturalists, not to mention Olympians.

82
percentage of mothers, in one study, who cite crime and safety concerns as factors for preventing their kids from playing outside.
(Contemporary Issues in Early Childhood, 2004)

38
percentage that violent victimization of children has dropped since 1975.
(Duke University Child Well Being Index, 2005)

🌀 Expert Opinion 🌀
Parenting Rules for a New World
By Dr. David Orr, professor of environmental studies, Oberlin College,
author of The Nature of Design: Ecology, Culture and
Human Intention

What will our children's children's children likely think about present child-raising practices? If they have the inclination and wherewithal, they will likely wonder about the depth of our affection for our children and our competence as parents. They will find it remarkable that we:

- risked the future of all children with both nuclear weapons and now climate change.
- exposed our children to poisons that undermined their physical, mental, and reproductive health.
- immersed our children in the artificial world of television, entertainment, and virtual reality, apparently without much thought to the toll that counterfeit reality would exact on their humanity.
- removed our children from direct contact with animals, farms, forests, and wild places, causing a kind of "nature deficit disorder," an incalculable loss of both spirit and competence.

What can we do to improve parenting? Most important, we must protect children and childhood, which means changing our priorities. As a society, that means such things as fewer shopping malls and more parks; less television and more family time; fewer roads and more trails. It means no child left behind . . . in every way. It means we must understand how to prepare them to live and flourish in the post–fossil fuel world. They need to know about solar energy, growing food, shelter, community building, and health. We must prepare them not only to survive in that new world but also to repair it. We should aim to foster and encourage physical and moral stamina, clarity of mind, and commitment to each other and to preserve their common humanity.

That goal requires that we, parents and teachers, foster a sense of hope along with the competence to act faithfully. Hope and competence include old and durable standards of decency, compassion, and foresight but now extended to all life for as far out as we can imagine. But hope grows out of the practical necessities to:

1. love our children thoughtfully and consistently.

2. slow the velocity of life by eating together, playing together, reading together, working together.

3. eat well, which means mostly local, organic, and unprocessed foods.

4. engage the natural world—more accurately, to enjoy a love affair with it. The natural world is not an abstraction . . . yet.

Step #7. Recruit the Kids

Since you're making all these changes to your home and habits mostly for your children, maybe all for them, why not involve them? Getting your kids to help—be it recycling, shopping for healthy food, or making DIY cleaning products and then marching around the house spritzing—brings with it all sorts of bonuses, beyond the nurturing of a healthier physical environment. The kids are infused with a feeling of accomplishment, of camaraderie (with family and planet both), of leadership. They become more aware of consequences and costs.

Make traditions. In the Northeast, my father said, one "tradition" was not turning on the heat until November first. I remember some mornings seeing my breath as I hopped out of bed, cold hands and feet while doing homework, hustling to keep warm—but my brothers and I were all proud we weren't "wasting" heat.

When you're engaging in the process of representative democracy, bring them in, too. It's an invaluable education and their voice, despite their inability to vote, carries weight. Color pages and have them write a statement; take a picture of them with a poster spelling out their concerns, like "Keep toxic chemicals out of my toys!" The humble truths spoken by children compel policy makers to attention. What adult wants to be shamed by a child?

There are more happy benefits to involving kids: When they chip in, you do less. Plus, it's time together. And it's fun.

Step #8. Calculate How Much Sense (Dollars) It Makes

While many people say they won't or can't go green/organic because of the expense, in fact you save money—lots—when you compute the savings over the course of the lifestyle change. Here are just a few areas where embracing a greener life provides economic benefit (the best way to persuade some skeptics):

Buy Energy Star–rated equipment. Maybe your less efficient model still does the job but each year you use an Energy Star dishwasher, refrigerator, or other big-ticket item you save significantly because of reduced energy cost—about $110 per year for a washing machine, $30 a year for a dishwasher or dehumidifier, $10 per year for a ceiling fan. (See energystar.gov for more price savings.) If you can't wait until your conventional machine dies, you may be eligible for a rebate for trading in your energy guzzler (fridge, air conditioner, etc.) for an Energy Star version. Ask your regional utility if they offer such a program.

Replace incandescents with compact fluorescent lightbulbs. Sure, the average CFL costs more than a comparable incandescent, but the CFL lasts five to seven times longer, saving you about twenty dollars per light over the course of the CFL's life. Looked at another way, if you changed five frequently used conventional bulbs in your house to CFLs, you'd save about twenty-five dollars per year. Considering that the average number of lights in an American home is forty-five(!), suddenly the larger up-front investment seems negligible.

Drive a hybrid car. Some doubt whether hybrid cars, with their higher price tag, can save money, but a recent study said unequivocally yes for every one of the twenty-two available hybrid models. You can get tax credits and lower insurance costs, plus a hybrid car is likelier to maintain its value after five years, compared to its nonhybrid cousin (an improvement of 5–15 percent). With oil hitting record highs seemingly every day, the savings reaped by drivers of hybrids are only increasing.

Consider smaller stuff. By building a smaller home, driving a smaller car, using the right wattage bulb rather than one brighter than you even want, you tax the environment and your bank account far less.

Finally, and perhaps most important, when you buy admittedly more expensive green products on a recurring basis (shampoo, organic produce, cleaning products), you reduce the risk of sickness, and the large financial outlay—often catastrophic outlay—that comes with that.

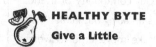 **HEALTHY BYTE**
Give a Little

At justgive.org, you can make donations securely, search for charitable organizations, research their histories, review their financials, and create a wish list of organizations for friends and family to support. There's even a kid's portal where little ones can learn about giving, and can choose charities.

If donating money is not an option, contact a charity you care about and ask what they need. Many organizations, particularly small community ones, have wish lists of simple items—printer paper, plants for the office, office furniture, etc.

Finally, when giving or investing, look for where your dollars will be matched—by your company or through state or federal credits.

Parentblog
When Your Other Half Is Greener

By Jessica Capshaw, actress, mom to Luke, wife of this book's author

Christopher likes to say that I'm a lighter shade of green than he is. And he's right, I am. It's not that I'm not environmentally aware—I was born in small-town Missouri surrounded by farmland, which is as green as it gets. But when it comes to environmental awareness there is no doubt about it, he knows more and practices more diligently to keep his, mine, and our lives as green as we can make them. When one person in a couple is more informed about any social or political or health issue that affects the decisions made at home, it's hard to say, *Okay, you do it your way and I'll do it mine.* Part of marriage, and of parenting, is learning to negotiate who gets to worry about what. And without a doubt, he governs over the "greenness" of our home.

People sometimes ask me, *How do you not flip out when your partner knows the health and hazards of everything you eat, put on your skin, let into your home?* My answer is, *I do flip out, but then I remember for every yin there is a yang and one of us has to be the skeptic.* Sometimes a new study or a new product will come out and our community of friends and family immediately react with, *I've got to stop doing this immediately* or *I have to use only this now!* But I like to take more time to weigh things, to understand the complete picture and not just react to a part of it. I remember once we had just come from doing our baby gift registry, and one of the things we'd registered for was a new European baby monitor. Christopher mentioned a study he had just read that suggested that cordless monitors could disrupt early sleep patterns. I was like, *What?* I couldn't believe it. Now I have to worry about monitors? And then I wanted to know everything about the study. *Who did it? What did they find? What monitors were tested?* Everything. That's where I get active, because I was not going to believe so quickly that something so accepted and necessary could be potentially harmful. I needed more information, and we did our research together. And yes, we have a baby monitor.

Then there were times when I was pregnant that Christopher would bring up new information or studies that pertained to my pregnancy. And sometimes that information was overwhelming—even scary to me—and I would say, *You know, actually, let's not talk about that right now.* And then sometimes the information felt empowering and enriching. It's a balance of information and timing. When to listen, learn, understand; and then knowing when to say when. I think the key is to acknowledge the rightness of each other's actions. To not shove information down each other's throats. It's all about delivery. And I've helped Christopher become better with the appropriateness of his timing.

When I see Christopher doing what he does, making a difference in the world and in our home—for instance, when we found out we were expecting he went through my medicine chest looking for beauty products containing unhealthy chemicals—I know it's actually right, and better for me and our son. Over the years it's become very instinctive to eat more organic food, to be more energy-conscious, and know which beauty products and which plastics contain unwanted ingredients so that we don't use them. When he suggests alternate options, he's being cautious and helpful, and I'm thankful for that.

In any area of life, that's what we need to do—get as much information as we can but also be true to who we are. In our case, Christopher is passionate about investigating, uncovering, and absorbing as much environmental and health information into our family's life as he can, and I'm happy to let him. It behooves me to learn from his expertise while not becoming completely overwhelmed by it. He checks everything in our house; I don't. He reads all these studies; I don't. I am light green and he is a dark and beautiful forest green. And I would say on any day of the week that my family is better for our individually distinctive shades.

Step #9. Keep the Faith

When pondering issues like your child's health and well-being, not to mention that of the planet he or she is inheriting, it's easy to feel lots of "d" things—distressed, dazed, dumbfounded, depressed. That's understandable, at least at first, but if you're to succeed at making real change in your home and world, then you need the right attitude—so flip over the "d" and instead be lots of "p" things:

- **Positive.** Optimism and hopefulness motivate you and those around you. Plus, to get someone to help you accomplish something, sweetness goes a long way.
- **Persistent.** If you can't get someone to listen, talk to someone else. If the solution you're offering isn't working, try Plan B. Don't give up.
- **Pragmatic.** Figure out if the outcome you're striving toward is achievable. Are you aiming too high? Are you operating under the assumption that everything will go as planned, and everyone will act reasonably? Is that realistic?
- **Patient.** Success is almost never immediate. People are busy; institutions and organizations have budgets and priorities to consider. Maybe it's best to pursue your goal at the start of next school year, or when your friend can join the effort, or after you complete a major project at work. It's great to get going the day before yesterday but patience is still a virtue.
- **(Full of) Perspective.** When making important changes—or being frustrated by the lack of progress in making them—it's easy to lose sight of things: the fight becomes everything, or all is lost if you haven't succeeded. It's vital to maintain the ability to step back (or to have someone you trust and love remind you to step back) and remember all the other things that matter.

 DIV

Throw a Party—Our Treat!

Call it the twenty-first-century Tupperware party: Invite friends over, open some (organic) wine, talk about how to protect kids' health and develop healthier environments, and send them home well-fed, well-informed, and revved up. Host a Healthy Home party and we'll help you out: Healthy Child will supply—free—a short, informational DVD narrated by Amy Brenneman, fact sheets, and green party favors such as literature and product samples from our green partners. (See healthychild.org for more details.) Here are some things to consider as you prep to promote a great cause while having fun.

Pick the venue. Tie it to a play date, block party, PTA meeting, open house at your school/child-care facility . . . or throw a party for no reason. Host it at home or in a park, rec center, or library.

Get the word out. Invite guests via online or phone; no paper, no waste.

Walk the talk. Exemplify your values at the party: Serve organic fruits and veggies; use real cups and plates; fill your home with a warm natural scent by putting herbs or spices in boiling water; print materials to share on recycled, PCF (processed chlorine-free) paper, and print on both sides. If you invite kids, make DIY play dough or gloop (see page 142), and provide nontoxic art supplies.

Share experiences. Invite guests to ask questions and talk about their own successes and struggles in creating healthy homes. Ask them if you can share their stories and concerns, in an e-mail or newsletter. Shared stories inspire others to act (and perhaps to throw their own Healthy Home parties).

Have fun. A party whose theme is reducing environmental threats to our children's health is not your normal beer blast, so try not to overwhelm guests with information to the point that they feel hopeless. Keep upbeat, focus on simple things we can all do that have an impact, and enjoy the festivities.

 ## Parentblog
Raising an Environmentalist
By Sheryl Crow, musician, activist

When my son Wyatt was three months old I was playing a concert in Toledo, so on my day off I took him to the zoo, a very beautiful old Victorian zoo with buildings from the turn of the century. At the polar bear exhibit, Wyatt's face lit up when he saw the baby polar bear stand up on its hind legs. It was amazing for me to watch the two of them connect—these living beings who share a planet. But I also felt panic and overwhelming sadness, knowing what's happening to polar bears, and the impact our environment is having on them and on us.

While I was on the global warming tour in 2007 I saw that panic was not just a grownup thing: Kids express their panic just as much, about environmental threats and dwindling opportunities. After all, they see the same images we adults see, read some of the same things we read. Yet I saw something else in them, something very hopeful: the birth of new activists. Kids don't just feel helplessness and panic but a sense of injustice, too. I sometimes think the thing that keeps adults from acting is cynicism, a belief that we *can't* really change things; we desensitize ourselves to the news; apathy puts us to sleep. And once you're asleep, you can't do anything.

Kids aren't like that. They don't have that cynicism in them, not yet anyway. They're awake to what's around them, so they can actually do something about it. We teach our kids all these ideals: Let's leave the Earth a better place than we found it; if you see something wrong, you can change it through action or education. Yet as we get older, we stop believing what we're saying. Kids, on the other hand, are motivated not just by what's in their heads but by what they actually see, like a baby polar bear. Kids are so acutely aware and smart, they will be the ones to motivate us, their parents, to change.

Step #10. Do Something

No one can do everything but everyone can do something. Stop, start, switch; make noise, boycott, volunteer, write a congressperson, choose, engage, speak up, learn. Join something established or begin something new. To give yourself the best shot to succeed with your proposed change, here are a few considerations:

Make deals with yourself. So maybe you won't give up all your incandescent bulbs or toss your old reliable of a non-Energy-Star-rated washing machine, and may be you love to eat steak and swordfish, or you take pleasure in washing your car by hand. We all have things we won't give up—and things we *will*. Figure out what changes and "deprivations" you can live with, and what you can't. Or at least find ways to improve situations where you indulge. Love long showers? Fine—but how about installing an inexpensive low-flow showerhead? Love wall-to-wall carpeting? Okay, but see if you can find an eco-sensible version without harmful glues. Life's a negotiation.

Make priorities. There are so many things to change, better make a list. Which ones can you accomplish quickly? Cheaply? Painlessly? Which ones are most critical for your family's health? Which can wait? It doesn't make sense to switch to organic peaches to reduce pesticide exposure, while continuing to spray your lawn with chemical pesticide.

Start small. Switching from conventional bedding, flooring, and furnishings on Monday to all-organic by Friday is laudable but unrealistic (or outside your budget). Set reasonable goals. Maybe start by swapping in organic sheets. See how they feel. Then maybe go for the organic mattress. Just as nothing slams the brakes on progress more than a sense that you've failed right at the start, nothing spurs progress like having milestones, now matter how small, that you've reached.

Pick one thing. Again, going all-out, while admirable, may not be the most efficient way to build a cleaner life. How about starting by changing cleaning products? Or testing and filtering the water? By seeing one issue through, you gain confidence to tackle the next, plus you get to check off an entire category, which translates to peace of mind.

Volunteer. Your time is valuable, to you *and* to others. Most organizations are flexible in how they engage volunteers. You could commit to a regular, long-term position (office work or community outreach), a short-term effort (event organizing), even just a few hours (envelope stuffing).

Something out there fits your schedule. Often, if you tell the organization of a specific area of interest and expertise, they'll find something you'll enjoy and be good at, too. Trust me: Nonprofits *love* volunteers.

Find your passion. It doesn't matter if it's an issue of local concern or global profundity. No one can do everything but everyone can do something.

ONE STEP BEYOND
Run for Office

You've remade your home but it doesn't feel like nearly enough; you want to remake your kids' park, school, neighborhood, country. Maybe it's time to work on a stump speech. With a seat on the school board, park board, neighborhood association, or even city council (or higher office), you've got a public forum for your vision and, more important, power over funds, and thus the influence to improve policies that affect kids' health.

Five Easy Steps for a Cleaner, Greener, Safer Home

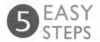

1. Manage Pests Safely.

Choose nontoxic lawn and garden products for insecticides, pesticides, weed killers, fertilizers, and flea/tick control. Remember to encourage good sanitation habits, such as washing hands after being outdoors and taking shoes off at the door.

2. Use Nontoxic Products.

Remember to read the labels and ask questions. USE products labeled NONTOXIC, CHLORINE-FREE, PHOSPHATE-FREE, NATURAL FRAGRANCE, PARABEN-FREE, HYPOALLERGENIC, VEGETABLE/BIO/WATER BASED, PETROLEUM-FREE, ORGANIC, LOW or ZERO VOC, RECYCLED or RECLAIMED, and FORMALDEHYDE-FREE. AVOID using products that say POISON, DANGER, WARNING, or CAUTION.

3. Clean Up Indoor Air.

Ventilate your home, especially the bedrooms and nursery, by simply opening windows. Change the filters in your air-conditioning and heating units—and the bag in your vacuum cleaner—to greatly improve indoor air quality. Sanitize and cleanse air with help from indoor plants and air purifiers with approved HEPA filters. Look for low VOC paints and stains. AVOID synthetic carpets when possible.

4. Shop Smart.

Eat organic fruits and vegetables when available. Make wise protein choices with meat, poultry, seafood, eggs and milk products from animals raised on vegetarian feed without hormones or antibiotics. AVOID foods high in sugar, high in fat, or highly processed, as well as fast foods.

5. Be Wise with Plastics.

Replace vinyl chew toys made of soft plastic, especially any labeled PVC, V, or #3. Opt for toys and books made with natural wood, cloth, or metal. AVOID using plastic containers and cling wrap in the microwave. Instead select reusable containers made of glass or ceramic (lead free). Choose safer plastics such as polyethylene (#1, #2, and #4) and polypropylene (#5). AVOID use of polycarbonate plastics for baby, and look for products that state NO PHTHALATES or NO BISPHENOL A (BPA).

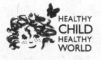 *Ensuring a healthy home for your children is of utmost importance. Healthy Child Healthy World helps us all learn about the opportunities we have to make simple, wise choices to create a healthy environment for our families to flourish.*

HEALTHY RESOURCES

Healthier, Nontoxic, Greener, Sustainable, Efficient,
Safer, Cleaner Products, Services, and
Informational Resources

Healthy Shopping and Learning

Air Quality

The Air Guys
In-home air assessments and
analysis.
indoorenvironmentcheck.com,
866-337-6653

Allergy Buyers Club
Air and water purifiers, dust mite
covers, vacuums, and bedding.
allergybuyersclub.com,
888-236-7231

Austin Air Purifiers
HEPA air filters for home, office,
and nursery.
austinairpurifiers.com, 866-300-3875

ClearFlite Air Purifiers
A wide range of products and expert
advice.
airpurifiers.com, 800-497-8263

RadonZone
Low-cost source of EPA-approved
radon testing kits and services.
radonzone.com, 866-992-3910

Art

**Art and Creative Materials Institute
(ACMI)**
A leading authority on nontoxic
art and creative materials,
founded in 1936. acminet.org,
781-293-4100

Budget Art Materials
Specializing in nontoxic and
environmentally friendly art supply
alternatives.
budgetartmaterials.com,
866-438-8080

Crayon Rocks
Coloring tools made of

renewable soybean wax and
tinted with natural mineral powders.
crayonrocks.net, 800-288-3363

EcoChoices EcoArtWorks
Environmentally safe crayons,
paints, papers, and supplies.
ecoartworks.com

Green Home
From soybean-based crayons to
recycled craft paper.
greenhome.com, 877-282-6400

Paporganics
Sustainable stationery and gift wrap.
paporganics.com, 800-340-4631

Baby Bedding and Crib Mattresses

Cotton Monkey
Organic cotton baby products.
cottonmonkey.com, 214-367-0719

Coyuchi, Inc.
Organic cottons sheets, baby
bedding, and towels.
coyuchiorganic.com, 888-418-8847

Hästens Beds
High quality, handmade beds from
natural materials for more than 150
years.
hastens.com

Mary Cordaro Collection
Healthy home products, including
crib mattresses and organic linens.
h3environmental.com, 818-766-1787

Naturepedic Organic Baby Mattress
"No compromise" eco-friendly
and organic crib mattresses and
bedding.
naturepedic.com, 800-917-3342

Pixel Organics
Infant bedding sets from 100%
organic cotton and 100%
regenerated fill.
pixelorganics.com, 213-746-0024

Baby Bottles

Born Free
Safer, non-BPA plastic baby bottles
and glass bottles.
newbornfree.com, 877-999-2676

Medela
BPA-free breast-feeding pumps,
bags, accessories, and storage sets.
medela.com, 800-435-8316

Think Baby Bottles
Nontoxic plastic and glass baby
bottles and sippy cups.
thinkbabybottles.com, 877-446-1616

Wee•go Glass Bottle
Safe and eco-friendly glass baby
bottles and products.
gobabylife.com, 415-339-0227

Baby/Child Care Products

Burt's Bees Herbal Insect Repellent
Natural oil blends that repel pests
without DEET.
burtsbees.com

California Baby
All-natural and sensitive line of bath and skin care for pregnancy and children.
californiababy.com, 877-576-2825

Earth Mama Angel Baby
Skin and body care products to support the birth process.
Toxin-free and vegan.
earthmamaangelbaby.com, 503-607-0607

Hippo and Turtle/Perfect Organics
Organic, vegan body care for babies and kids. Free of parabens and synthetic fragrance.
hippoandturtle.com, 800-653-1078

LiceMeister
The only comb endorsed by the National Pediculosis Association.
headlice.org/licemeister, 866-323-5465 ext. 8065

Terressentials
Hand-crafted, 100% certified organic personal care products.
terressentials.com

Weleda
Natural baby care with healing botanicals.
usa.weleda.com, 800-241-1030

Baby Clothing

BabySoy
Designer soybean fiber baby clothes and products.
babysoyusa.com, 888-769-7638

Bamboosa
Naturally antimicrobial and hypoallergenic bamboo fiber clothing and products.
bamboosa.com, 800-673-8461

Better For Babies
Cloth diapers, organic wool, pregnancy, and cosleeping info and products.
betterforbabies.com, 877-303-4050

Eco-Wise
Baby clothes, baby care products, slings, and more.
ecowise.com, 512-326-4474

Green Babies
U.S.-made certified organic cotton clothing for babies and kids.
greenbabies.com, 800-603-7508

Hanna Andersson
A Swedish heritage line of earth-friendly clothing for families.
hannaandersson.com, 800-222-0544

Kate Quinn Organics
Clothing, bedding, and linens from 100% certified organic cotton.
katequinnorganics.com, 877-760-2997

Kee-Ka, Inc.
Eco-chic apparel and gifts.
kee-ka.com, 718-302-9665

Kid Bean
Earth-friendly, labor-friendly, vegan
products for your family.
kidbean.com, 866-253-0009

Nui Organics
Certified organic merino wool
clothing.
nuiorganics.com, 888-823-6480

Positively Organic
Bright and bold organic cotton
clothing.
positively-organic.com,
646-286-5966

Pure Beginnings
Organic cotton clothing and
bedding, plus organic skin care.
purebeginnings.com,
866-787-2229

Sage Creek Naturals
Eco-friendly dyed, organic cotton
baby bedding, and layette.
sagecreeknaturals.com,
877-513-2183

Speesees
Organic, fair-trade cotton kids'
clothing and clothing donation
programs.
speesees.com, 415-552-5808

Under the Nile
100% organic cotton apparel,
accessories, toys, blankets, and
diapers.
underthenile.com,
800-710-1264

Baby Products: Retail/Online

Better for Babies
Natural and organic baby products.
betterforbabies.com, 877-303-4050

Branch Home
Eco-sensitive, high-design home
goods, furnishings, and kids' items.
branchhome.com, 415-341-1824

Eco Mall
Portal for thousands of green,
eco-friendly products and services.
ecomall.com

Giggle
A wide selection of all the
essentials for your "healthy, happy
baby."
egiggle.com, 800-495-8577

The Little Seed
L.A. children's boutique carrying
eco-friendly and organic products.
thelittleseed.com, 323-462-4441

Maple Grace
High-quality, organic, nontoxic
products for newborns, toddlers,
and home.
maplegrace.com,
877-432-6248

Our Green House
Clean and healthy home products.
ourgreenhouse.com, 203-364-1484

Pur Bébé
Natural and organic baby boutique.
purbebe.com, 877-850-3313

Sage Baby
Eco-friendly baby and nursery
boutique.
sagebabynyc.com, 917-930-1852

Tiny Birds Organics
Environmentally friendly kids'
products store.
tinybirdsorganics.com

Baby Showers and Gifts

Organic Bouquet
A certified organic flower arranging
company.
organicbouquet.com,
877-899-2468

Pure Home Products
Eco-friendly online boutique with
green registry for baby showers and
gift giving.
purehomeproducts.com,
877-432-6248

Backyard Play

CedarWorks
Wooden swing sets free of chemical
treatments, paints, or stains.
cedarworks.com, 800-462-3327

ChildLife
Play systems made with cedar,
ladder system, and maple climbing
rungs.
childlife.com, 800-467-9464

The Natural Playgrounds Company
Designers of innovative,

eco-sensitive, equipment-free
natural playgrounds.
naturalplaygrounds.com,
888-290-8405

Playmart Playgrounds
Makers of playground equipment
from Recycled Structural Plastic
(RSP) posts, decks, and railings.
playmart.com, 800-940-7529

Progressive Design Playgrounds
Environmentally friendly playground
equipment from 100% recycled
plastic.
pdplay.com, 800-585-3131

Safe Sand Company
Chemically free "safe" sand for your
sandbox.
safesand.com, 415-971-1776

Bath

Earthsake
Bathroom products and bedding
made of organic cotton, bamboo,
and wool.
earthsake.com, 877-268-1026

Green Sage Store
Organic cotton towels and robes and
sustainable bathroom accessories.
greensage.com/bath.html,
415-453-7915

Happy Planet
Shower curtains, linens, towels, bath
mats from quality sustainable
materials.

ahappyplanet.com,
800-811-3213

Raw Ganique
Organic cotton, linen, and hemp
products for bath and home.
rawganique.com, 877-729-4367

Beauty/Personal Care

Aubrey Organics
Natural hair and skin care products
free of synthetics and
petrochemicals.
aubreyorganics.com,
800-282-7394

Avalon Organics
Bath, body and baby care
products made with natural plant
botanicals.
avalonorganics.com, 800-227-5120

Aveda
Makeup, hair, and skin care products
from organic, plant-based, and
mineral ingredients.
aveda.com, 800-644-4831

Crystal Body Deodorant
The Environmental Working Group
ranks The Crystal as the #1 safest
deodorant.
thecrystal.com, 800-829-7625

Dr. Hauschka
Holistic skin care using ecological
methods of growing and sourcing
ingredients.
drhauschka.com, 800-247-9907

EcoColors
Nontoxic hair color line; great choice
for chemical sensitivity and
pregnancy.
ecocolors.net, 877-852-4515

Giovanni Organic Hair Care
Hair and skin care products with
blends of certified organic
botanicals.
giovannicosmetics.com,
310-952-9960

Glad Rags
An assortment of menstrual
products made with organic
cotton.
gladrags.com, 800-799-4523

John Masters Organics
Hair and skin care products with no
artificial colorings or fragrances.
johnmasters.com, 212-343-9590

Nature's Gate
Natural products from baby care to
deodorants, oral care, and acne
treatments.
natures-gate.com, 800-327-2012

Origins Organics
Skin, body, and hair care products
certified by USDA National Organic
Program.
originsorganics.com

The Organic Pharmacy
One-stop shop for organic lotions
and potions.
theorganicpharmacy.com

Pangea Organics
Skin and body care products using
plant essences with vitamins,
minerals, and essential oils.
pangeaorganics.com, 877-679-5854

Perfect Organics
Organic, vegan personal care
products.
perfectorganics.com, 800-653-1078

Suki's Naturals
100% natural skin care products.
sukisnaturals.com, 888-858-7854

Weleda
Complementary medicine and
cosmetics with no synthetic
preservatives.
usa.weleda.com, 800-241-1030

Bedding and Bath

Anna Sova
Luxury organic Italian linens with
eco-safe cotton bleaching, dyeing,
and finishing.
annasova.com, 877-326-7682

Coyuchi
Organic bath and baby products,
cotton bedding and blankets.
coyuchi.com, 888-418-8847

EcoChoices
Natural bedding and mattresses
from organic cotton, pure-grow
wool, hemp, and natural latex.
ecobedroom.com, 626-969-3707

Gaiam
Affordable beautiful organic cotton
bedding, plus other green lifestyle
products.
gaiam.com, 877-989-6321

Green Nest
Organic bedding, HEPA filters,
towels, linens, and more.
greennest.com, 888-473-6466

Green Sleep
Organic mattresses, pads, pillows,
and frame systems.
greensleep.com, 888-413-4442

Hästens Beds
High-quality handmade Swedish
beds from natural materials for more
than 150 years.
hastens.com

LifeKind
A full line of certified organic
bedding products.
lifekind.com, 800-284-4983

Loop Organic
Certified organic cotton sheets and
towels.
looporganic.com, 800-987-5667

Natura
Mattresses, bedding, pillows, and
crib sets from natural latex and
organic wool.
naturaworld.com, 888-628-8723

The Organic Mattress Store
Online store of nontoxic and

organic bedding, pillows, and mattresses.
organicmattressstore.com, 866-246-9866

Vivètique
Maker of natural and organic bedding and mattresses.
vivetique.com, 800-365-6563

Carbon Offsetting

LiveNeutral
A nonprofit that calculates your carbon emissions to neutralize your carbon footprint.
liveneutral.org, 415-695-2355

Terrapass
Balance your carbon impact for your car, plane flights, powering your home, and beyond.
terrapass.com/hchw, 877-210-9581

Cleaning Products and Supplies

Biokleen
Produce Wash removes chemical sprays, waxes, and soils.
biokleen.com, 800-240-5536

Dr. Bronner's Magic Soaps
For more than fifty years, certified organic Castile soap with essential oils and no additives.
drbronners.com, 877-786-3649

Ecover
Ecological and economic dish-washing and cleaning products.
ecover.com, 800-449-4925

Method
enviro-friendly cleaning for the entire home.
methodhome.com, 866-963-8463

Mountain Green
Synthetic-free and hypoallergenic soy-based dryer sheets.
mountaingreen.biz, 866-686-4733

Restore Oven Cleaner
A nontoxic oven cleaner.
restoreproducts.com, 612-331-5979

Seventh Generation
The industry leader in creating house-hold and personal care products.
seventhgeneration.com, 800-456-1191

Shaklee
Since 1960, makers of the first biodegradable household cleaners.
shaklee.com, 800-670-6251

Starfiber
Microfiber cleaning cloths and mops.
starfibers.com, 562-663-1730

Clothing and Gear (Adult)

Blue Canoe
Adult organic cotton clothing, yoga apparel, casual clothing, and lingerie.
bluecanoe.com, 888-923-1373

GreenLoop
Clothing and accessories by
eco-conscious companies.
thegreenloop.com, 503-236-3999

H&M
Stylish, affordable clothing, some
using organic cotton and vegetable
dyes.
hm.com, 212-564-9922

Linda Loudermilk
Women's and baby clothing made of
sasawashi, bamboo, sea cell, soy, and
other self-sustaining plants.
lindaloudermilk.com,
323-233-8111

Nau
Clothing from enviro-friendly fabric
with functional design.
nau.com, 877-454-5628

Patagonia
Eco-minded utilitarian clothing.
patagonia.com, 800-638-6464

Rickshaw Bagworks, Inc.
Planet-conscious messenger bags,
packs, and cases for urban living.
rickshawbags.com,
415-904-8368

Zooey Tees
Organic cotton and bamboo
T-shirts that make a statement.
Zooey generously donates to
HCHW.
zooeytees.com/green,
888-360-7987

Construction and Remodeling

CARPETS / RUGS
Carpet America Recovery Effort
Carpet reclamation for recycled
content products.
carpetrecovery.org

Earth Weave
100% natural wool carpet—no
mothproofing or stain protections
with biodegradable adhesives.
earthweave.com, 706-278-8200

Interface Flor Carpet Tiles
Made from recycled or renewable
resources.
flor.com, 866-281-3567

Nature's Carpet
100% pure wool, ultralow toxicity
carpet filters.
naturescarpet.com, 800-667-5001

Shaw's Green Edge (Eco Worx Carpet)
Recycled content, low-VOC, Cradle-
to-Cradle designed carpet and tiles.
shawgreenedge.com

FLOORING
Duro-Design
Bamboo, cork, engineered oak, and
eucalyptus coupled with low-VOC
finishing systems.
duro-design.com, 888-528-8518

EcoTimber
Sustainable and reclaimed wood
flooring made without toxic
adhesives and additives.

ecotimber.com,
415-258-8454

Expanko
Cork flooring and recycled rubber.
expanko.com, 800-345-6202

Forbo Marmoleum
Healthy, hygienic flooring solutions
made with natural ingredients.
themarmoleumstore.com,
800-842-7839

GreenFloors
Catalog of environmentally friendly
flooring and recycled carpeting.
greenfloors.com, 703-352-8300

Natural Cork
Cork floors that are environmentally
sustainable and nontoxic.
Naturalcork.com, 800-404-2675

Teragren
Bamboo flooring, panels, and
veneers harvested sustainably.
teragren.com, 800-929-6333

GENERAL REMODELING MATERIALS
Bonded Logic
Natural cotton fiber insulation from
recycled denim.
bondedlogic.com, 480-812-9114

Ecohaus
Products, health and environmental
information and how-to's.
environmentalhomecenter.com,
800-281-9785

Environmental Depot
Green building and renovation
supplies for commercial and
residential applications.
environmentaldepot.com,
800-238-5008

Green Building Supply
Hundreds of name-brand products.
greenbuildingsupply.com,
800-405-0222

Greenhome
Catalog of green products and
services.
greenhome.com, 415-282-6400

Modern Green Living
Green residential developments and
links to green professionals.
moderngreenliving.com,
866-848-2840

Plan•It Hardware
Green it yourself with
environmentally friendly hardware
supplies.
planithardware.com, 877-359-9914

TerraMai
Reclaimed wood for flooring,
lumber, beams and timber, decking,
siding, and paneling.
terramai.com, 800-220-9062

INFORMATIONAL SITES
Green Building
All about green building.
greenbuilding.com, 303-444-7044

Green Building Blocks
Listings of environmentally sound
building and remodeling products.
greenbuildingblocks.com

Green Home Building
Information on sustainable
architecture and natural building.
greenhomebuilding.com

Healthy House Institute
Information for creating healthier
homes.
healthyhouseinstitute.com,
208-938-3137

PAINTS AND PLASTERS
AFM
Environmentally responsible paints,
stains, finishes, sealers.
safecoatpaint.com, 800-239-0321

American Clay
Natural clays, recycled and
reclaimed aggregates, in natural
pigments.
americanclay.com, 866-404-1634

Anna Sova
Healthy wall finishes with no VOCs,
and made with 99% food-grade
ingredients.
annasova.com, 877-326-7682

Auro
Natural interior and exterior paints,
primers, sealer, stains, varnishes,
adhesives.
aurousa.com, 888-302-9352

Bioshield
Nontoxic wood stains, paints,
finishes, primers, thinners,
adhesives, cleaners, floor care
products.
bioshieldpaint.com, 800-621-2591

Yolo Colorhouse
Environmentally responsible paint
with a natural palette.
yolocolorhouse.com, 877-493-8275

PAINT REMOVER
Silent Paint Remover
Remove paint and varnish from
wood with gentle infrared heat.
silentpaintremover.com,
585-924-8070

Soy Clean
Strippers, stains, and sealers made
from soybeans.
soyclean.biz, 641-522-9559

Cosmetics

Bare Escentuals
Mineral makeup with 100% natural
formula.
bareescentuals.com, 800-227-3990

CARE from Stella McCartney
Certified organic ingredients with
essential nutrients to keep skin
healthy.
stellamccartneycare.com

Jane Iredale
Micronized minerals cosmetics

made without fillers and binders.
janeiredale.com, 800-762-1132

Josie Maran
Palette of multi-use makeup with natural/organic ingredients and biodegradable packaging.
josiemarancosmetics.com, 866-292-2304

Diapers

gDiapers
Not cloth and not disposable; washable cover and a flushable insert.
gdiapers.com, 866-553-5874

Heavenly Organic Cloth Diapers
100% organic cloth diapers, diaper covers, diapering accessories.
heavenlyorganic.com, 800-562-9074

Seventh Generation Diapers
Chlorine-free materials and absorbent polymers.
seventhgeneration.com, 802-658-3773

Tushies Diapers
Disposable diapers with certified nonchlorine-bleached wood pulp blended with cotton.
tushies.com, 800-344-6379

Food

CleanFish
Seafood from artisans who cultivate and harvest carefully.

cleanfish.com, 877-425-6374

Contessa Premium Foods
Environmentally responsible seafood and "green cuisine."
contessa.com

Earthbound Farm
Growers of certified organic produce with more than 100 varieties of salads and produce.
earthboundfarm.com, 800-690-3200

Eat Well Guide
Wholesome, sustainable food in the United States and Canada.
eatwellguide.org, 212-991-1858

Horizon Organics
Everything healthy and organic in the dairy department for your little ones.
horizonorganic.com

Local Harvest
Find farmers' markets, family farms, and other sources of sustainably grown food in your area.
localharvest.org, 831-475-8150

LUNA Bar
100% natural women's nutrition bar made with 70% USDA certified organic ingredients.
lunabar.com, 800-586-2227

Natural Food Coop Directory
Resource for natural food coops and locations near you.
coopdirectory.org, 651-774-9189

New Chapter Prenatal Vitamins
Organic probiotic whole-food
prenatal vitamin that promotes
stamina.
newchapter.info,
800-543-7279

Newman's Own Organics
Organic food with a focus on the
kinds of products we loved as kids.
newmansownorganics.com

NUI Kid Water
Low-sugar beverage packed with
vitamins, green tea, and nine high
antioxidant fruits.
nuiwater.com, 866-504-6684

Organic Valley Farms
100% organic milk, cheese, butter,
eggs, juice, soy beverages, produce,
meats.
organicvalley.coop, 888-444-6455

Sommers Organic
Family business providing organic
meats free of pesticides, antibiotics,
and hormones.
sommersorganic.com, 877-377-9797

Whole Foods Market
World's leading natural and organic
supermarket.
wholefoods.com, 866-936-2255

Wild Planet
Wild seafood from sustainable
fisheries.
1wildplanet.com,
800-998-9946

BABY FOOD AND FORMULA
Baby's Only Formula
Natural and organic soy formula,
dairy formula, with oral electrolytes,
DHA fatty acids, and probiotics.
naturesone.com, 888-227-7122

Bohemian Baby
Organic baby foods.
bohemian-baby.com,
800-708-7605 ext. 85

Happy Baby
Organic baby meals with 100%
natural ingredients.
happybabyfood.com

Homemade Baby
Baby food made fresh daily with
wholesome family recipes.
homemadebaby.com,
800-854-8507

Plum Organics
Organic baby food flash-frozen to
lock in flavor, freshness, and
nutrients.
plumorganics.com

Tasty Baby
Organic foods grown without toxic
pesticides and fertilizers, and
minimally processed.
tastybaby.com, 866-588-8278

Furniture—Home and Baby

ABC Carpet and Home
Eco-friendly products and
furnishings with sustainability

and global awareness in mind.
abchome.com, 212-473-3000

Branch Home
Environmentally sensitive home
goods, furnishings, and kids' items.
branchhome.com, 415-341-1824

Celery Furniture
Modern children's furniture made
with bamboo, nontoxic adhesives,
and 100% recycled fiberboard.
celeryfurniture.com, 888-556-7165

Environment Furniture
Reclaimed, recycled, and sustainable
wood furniture collection.
environment-furniture.com,
323-935-1330

Greener Lifestyles
Eco-friendly, 100% natural, and fair-
trade products.
greenerlifestyles.com, 888-220-6020

IKEA
Quality home furnishing products,
manufactured by environmentally
sensitive suppliers.
ikea.com, 800-434-4532

Nest
Modern, environmentally friendly
children's furnishings.
nestplease.com, 413-467-2086

Q Collection Junior
Line of healthy, eco-friendly
children's furniture and bedding.
qcollectionjunior.com, 800-775-0994

Spring
Green products for a healthy home.
astorecalledspring.com, 415-673-2065

2Modern
Featuring reclaimed wood, recycled
parts, and fair-trade pieces.
2modern.com, 888-222-4410

The Wooden Duck
Recycled wood furniture from
Indonesia, Europe, and China.
thewoodenduck.com, 510-848-3575

VivaTerra
Eco-retailer of home furnishings,
kitchen, dining, bath, and bedding
products.
vivaterra.com, 800-233-6011

Vivavi
Eco-friendly furniture and home
design center.
vivavi.com, 866-848-2840

Garden and Lawn

Arbico Organics
Online-only supplier of organic
products, test kits, and natural pest
control.
arbico-organics.com, 800-827-2847

Clean Air Gardening
Environmentally friendly lawn and
garden supplies.
cleanairgardening.com, 214-819-9500

The Dandelion Terminator
Removes dandelions and other

broadleaf weeds.
dlt100.com

EcoSmart
Nontoxic, organic insecticides
effective on a wide range of bugs while
keeping your family and pets safe.
buyecosmart.com, 877-723-3545

Extremely Green Gardening Company
Products for organic lawn, soil, and
garden care.
extremelygreen.com, 781-878-5397

Fertrell WeedBan
Weed control from a corn syrup
by-product.
fertrell.com, 717-367-1566

Gardens Alive!
Environmentally responsible lawn/
soil/plant care and insect control
products.
gardensalive.com, 513-354-1482

Hound Dog
Backyard tools including the Weed
Hound, Bulb Hound, Edge Hound,
and aerator.
hound-dog.com, 800-393-1846

Naturalawn of America
Environmentally sound lawn care.
naturalawn.com, 301-694-5440

**Peaceful Valley Farm and
Garden Supply**
For indoor plants, organic garden, or
lawn.
groworganic.com, 888-784-1722

Pharm Solutions, Inc.
Organic solutions—soap and
essential oils—for weed and insect
control.
organicpesticides.com, 805-927-7400

Seeds of Change
Organically grown vegetable, flower
and herb seeds, plus books, tools,
and more.
seedsofchange.com, 888-762-7333

TerraCycle
Organic products and fertilizers
made from plant wastes.
terracycle.net, 609-393-4252

Home Safety Test Kits

Homax Household Lead Test Kit
Test home products; simple-to-
understand results.
leadtesttoys.com

Hybrivet Systems
Easy test solutions for heavy
metals.
leadcheck.com, 800-262-5323

Watersafe
All-in-one kit to check water at home.
healthhometest.com, 877-275-7613

Housewares

COOKWARE
Calphalon
Cookware, cutlery, bakeware, and
kitchen tools.
calphalon.com, 800-809-7267

GreenPan
Ceramic, nontoxic, nonstick coated cookware.
green-pan.com

Lodge Cookware
Cast-iron bakeware, skillets, fryers, grill pans, griddles, Dutch ovens, and more.
castironcookware.com

DISPOSABLE DISHWARE
Biodegradable Store
Food containers, plates, bowls, utensils, cups, napkins, and more made from recycled paper.
biodegradablestore.com,
303-449-1876

Cereplast
Plastics made from corn, wheat, tapioca, and potato starches.
cereplast.com, 310-676-5000

EarthShell
Compostable plates, cups, cutlery, and food storage containers from fully biodegradable materials.
earthshell.com, 866-387-3233

Green Feet
Eco-home store with disposable dishware made from recycled and sugar-based plastics.
greenfeet.com, 888-562-8873

Preserve Kitchen
Sturdy plates, cutlery, and tumblers that can be reused; made from 100% recycled plastic.
recycline.com, 888-354-7296

Royal Chinet
Natural pulp fiber tableware; recyclable and compostable.
royalchinet.ca, 877-425-3462

FOOD STORAGE
Anchor Hocking Glassware
Glass containers—safer alternatives to plastic food storage.
anchorhocking.com,
800-562-7511 ext. 2478

BioBag
Made of GMO-free cornstarch and 100% biodegradable, in a variety of kitchen and household sizes.
biobagusa.com, 727-789-1646

Diamant Food Wrap
Non-PVC stretch food wrap containing no plasticizers or chlorine; completely recyclable.
diamantfilm.com,
905-752-0220

Fresh Baby
Food trays designed to simplify feedings and reduce waste of baby food and breast milk.
freshbaby.com, 866-403-7374

Pyrex
Glass prepware, bakeware, cookware, serving, and storage.
pyrexware.com,
800-999-3436

Lighting

American Scientific Lighting
Largest line of energy-efficient fixtures in the United States.
asllighting.com, 800-369-1101

Solatube
Reflective tubing material that transfers up to five times more daylight to your indoor spaces.
solatube.com, 888-765-2882

Sunalux
Designs and manufactures healthy, full-spectrum lighting.
sunalux.com, 800-339-9572

Mosquito Repellent

Bite Blocker
#1 DEET alternative.
biteblocker.com, 888-270-5721

Repel
Safe and effective against mosquitoes, deer ticks, and no-see-ums for up to six hours.
repel.com, 800-332-5553

Pest Control

Battle
Safe, effective, nontoxic, odorless pest control made from limestone.
battlethosebugs.com, 800-785-7903

Bugs 'R' Done
Made with pure orange peel extract; safe for use around kids and animals.
bugsrdone.com, 561-742-0080

Garden Supply
Organic gardening supplies for sustainable agriculture and home gardens.
groworganic.com, 888-784-1722

Gardens Alive!
Products for lawn/soil/plant care, plus insect and animal pest control.
gardensalive.com, 513-354-1483

Safe Solutions, Inc.
Nontoxic household products—organic, sustainable, biodegradable.
safesolutionsinc.com, 888-443-8738

Pet Supplies

BioBag USA
100% biodegradable, compostable poop bags.
biobagusa.com, 727-789-1646

Biocontrol Network
Natural pet care products, including flea trap.
biconet.com/pets, 615-370-4301

CityCats.biz
Organic catnip, cat grass, kitty and cat grass growing kits, cat food, more.
citycats.biz, 406-755-8690

DoggyArchy
Pesticide-free hemp bedding without harmful substances.
doggyarchy.com

Great Green Pets
Blog for the green pet owner.
greatgreenpet.com

Green Pets
All-natural, holistic dog, cat, and
other pet food, supplies, and
equipment.
greenpets.com, 202-986-7907

Mojo-D
Moisturizing, pest-repellent organic
dog shampoo.
greenearthgoods.net, 301-916-2035

Natura Pet Foods
Made with meats, whole grains,
fresh fruits, and vegetables.
naturapet.com, 800-532-7261

Only Natural Pet Store
Holistic pet health products.
onlynaturalpet.com, 888-937-6677

Organic and Nature
Naturally remove pet stains
and odors.
organicandnature.com,
877-520-5433

Safe Paw
Salt-free ice melter, nontoxic for
kids, pets, and water systems.
safepaw.com, 800-783-7841

SwheatScoop
Use wheat (and no chemicals) to
eliminate odor of cat litter.
swheatscoop.com, 800-794-3287

Vermont Soap Pet Shampoo
First USDA certified organic pet
shampoo.
vermontsoap.com/petwash.shtml,
866-762-7482

Renewable Energy

Green Mountain Energy Company
Provides "clean" energy and carbon
offsetting.
greenmountain.com, 866-785-4668

NativeEnergy
Certified renewable energy credits
for farmer-owned, community-based
projects.
nativeenergy.com, 800-924-6826

Reuse and Recycle

Baby Buggy
Nonprofit provides families in need
with donated infant equipment,
clothing, and products (New York
City).
babybuggy.org, 212-736-1777

Baby 2 Baby
Nonprofit gives baby/kids' gear
and clothing to needy families
(Los Angeles).
baby2baby.org, 323-933-2229

Craigslist
Local classifieds and forums for 450
cities worldwide; community-
moderated, largely free.
craigslist.org

Earth 911
Where and what to recycle, and who takes your hazardous waste.
earth911.org, 800-253-2687

eBay Giving Works
List items and donate a portion of final sale price.
givingworks.ebay.com/sell

Freecycle
Grassroots network giving (and getting) stuff for free in their own towns.
freecycle.org

National Recycling Coalition
Who's in charge of your community's recycling; what they'll take.
nrc-recycle.org, 202-789-1430

Stuff Ya Don't Want
To discard stuff that's just lying around.
stuffyadontwant.com

The Thrift Shopper
For thrift shopping needs.
thethriftshopper.com, 321-441-4131

School Lunches

Laptop Lunches
Nontoxic food containers for school lunches.
laptoplunches.com, 831-457-0301

Organic Lunch box
A resource for creating an organic lunch box for kids.

drgreene.org,
925-964-1793

Reusablebags.com
Shopping, grocery, and lunch bags that consider durability, value, ecological impact.
reusablebags.com, 888-707-3873

Sunscreen

Avalon Organics
Unscented sunscreen cream made with organic jojoba and sunflower oils.
avalonorganics.com, 800-227-5120

Aveeno
Sun block lotion SPF 45 especially for baby skin.
aveeno.com, 877-298-2525

Baby Blanket
Sun block products including zinc stick, scalp spray, body lotion, body spray.
babyblanketsuncare.com,
508-679-1941

Toys

Beyond Learning
Educational games made from FSC-certified papers with soy-based inks.
beyond-learning.com, 310-826-7409

Bioviva
Sustainable games from completely recycled paper, nontoxic vegetable ink, and zero glue.
bioviva.com/us

Crispina Fuchsia
Ragamuffins—soft, unique toys from
recycled wool sweaters.
crispina.com, 800-824-1143

Gifted Grasshopper
Book bags, party favor gift bags,
recommended reading lists.
giftedgrasshopperchildrensbooks.
com, 888-310-5745

Kenana Knitters
Toys from natural-plant dyed wools,
handmade by Kenyan women.
kenanausa.com, 800-336-3553

NaturalPlay.com
Nontoxic, wooden, natural games
that encourage interaction with
nature.
naturalplay.com, 608-637-3989

Nova
Natural toys, crafts, blocks, puzzles,
trains, playhouses.
novanatural.com, 877-668-2111

Oompa Toys
Wooden toys, baby toys, educational
toys, jewelry, bags, children's room
décor items.
oompa.com, 888-825-4109

Playstore Toys
Wooden toys; low environmental
impact.
playstoretoys.com, 877-876-1111

Tree Blocks
Wooden toys, blocks, tree houses,

dollhouses, learning-oriented
products.
treeblocks.com, 800-873-4960

Vacuum Cleaners

Bissell
"Healthy Home" bagless vacuum
with HEPA filtration.
bissell.com, 800-237-7691

Dyson
"DC" vacuums with lifetime HEPA
filtration; "asthma-friendly."
dyson.com, 866-693-9766

Miele
Vacuums with "Super Air Clean
Filters," high energy efficiency.
mielevacuums.com, 800-843-7231

Water

Bricor
Vacuum flow technology for low-flow
showerheads.
bricor.com, 830-624-7228

Caroma Dual-Flush Toilet
Two-button dual flush system, reduces
water usage by up to two-thirds.
caromausa.com, 800-605-4218

Filter Water
Water filtration products, lab-tested
and certified.
filterwater.com, 800-439-0263

Green Earth Waterless Car Wash
Waterless spray—biodegradable,

dye- and VOC-free.
greenearthcarwash.com,
310-215-3133

Pedal Valve Hands-Free Faucet
Foot valve for faucets, reduces
consumption.
pedalvalve.com, 800-431-3668

Oxygenics
Self-pressurizing, low-flow
showerhead.
oxygenics.com, 800-344-3242

Water Bottles

Klean Kanteen
Reusable, lightweight stainless steel
canteen.
kleankanteen.com, 530-345-3275

Sigg
Environmentally safe aluminum
bottles from Switzerland.
sigg.com, 203-321-1218

Thinksport Bottles
Stylized, nontoxic stainless steel
bottles.
thinksportbottles.com,
877-446-1616

Water Filtraton Certification

**NSF—The Public Health and Safety
Company**
Nonprofit that certifies products and
writes standards for food, water, and
consumer goods.
nsf.org, 800-673-6275

**Underwriter Laboratories Water
Quality Services**
Water testing and certifying for
entities that need to be compliant.
ul.com/water, 877-854-3577

Water Quality Association
Research water and find water
professionals.
wqa.org, 630-505-0160

NGOs and Groups

Alliance to Save Energy
Nonprofit, makes policy to promote
energy efficiency.
ase.org, 202-857-0666

American Lung Association
Fighting lung disease, with emphasis
on asthma, tobacco control,
environmental health.
lungusa.org, 800-586-4872

Beyond Pesticides
Resources about pesticides and
nontoxic alternatives.
beyondpesticides.org,
202-543-5450

Breast Cancer Fund
For breast cancer prevention,
including environmentally caused.
breastcancerfund.org, 415-346-8223

CERES
Investor coalition for improving
corporate environmental, social, and
governance practices.
ceres.org, 617-247-0700

Co-op America
Harnessing the economic power of
businesses and consumers for
greener business practices,
sustainability.
coopamerica.org, 800-584-7336

The Edible Schoolyard
A nonprofit for providing urban
public school students a chance to
learn about organic gardening.
edibleschoolyard.org, 510-558-1335

EnviroLink
Resources on the environment.
envirolink.org

Environmental Defense
Partners with corporations to
address environmental concerns.
environmentaldefense.org,
800-684-3322

Environmental Media Association
Mobilizes the entertainment
industry to educate and inspire
action.
ema-online.org, 310-446-6244

Environmental Working Group
Research organization, informs the
public on health and environmental
issues.
ewg.org, 202-667-6982

Friends of the Earth
U.S. arm of an international
grassroots network, for
environmental causes.
foe.org, 877-843-8687

Global Green USA
Addresses climate change; weapons
of mass destruction; clean, safe
water.
globalgreen.org, 310-581-2700

Greenguard Environmental Institute
Seeks to establish acceptable indoor
air quality standards for products,
environments, buildings.
greenguard.org, 800-427-9681

Greenpeace
Focused on environmental change
affecting oceans and land.
greenpeace.org, 800-326-0959

Health Care Without Harm
Focused on the health-care sector
and its ecological sustainability.
noharm.org/us, 703-243-0056

Healthy Schools Network
Education, coalition building, and
advocacy regarding healthy schools.
healthyschools.org,
518-462-0632

Kids for Saving Earth
Providing environmental education
curriculum for all ages.
kidsforsavingearth.org,
763-559-1234

League of Conservation Voters
Bipartisan work to educate voters
and win elections deemed good for
the environment.
lcv.org, 202-785-8683

National Center for Bicycling and Walking
Community planning, designing, and managing, to ensure biking and walking.
bikewalk.org, 301-656-4220

Natural Resources Defense Council
Using law and science to protect the environment.
nrdc.org, 212-727-2700

Oceana
Protecting oceans; education about issues for protection and restoration.
oceana.org, 877-762-3262

1% for the Planet
Businesses donate 1% of yearly sales to environmental groups worldwide.
onepercentfortheplanet.org, 978-462-5353

Organic Consumers Association
Organic rights, food safety, fair trade, and social justice.
organicconsumers.org, 218-226-4164

Public Interest Research Groups
The federation of PIRGs; environmental efforts.
uspirg.org, 202-546-9707

SafeLawns
A nonprofit for promoting natural lawn care and grounds maintenance.
safelawns.org, 800-251-1784

Sierra Club
Explore, enjoy, and protect the planet.
sierraclub.org, 415-977-5500

The Trust for Public Land
Conserving land to be (or remain) parks, community gardens, historic sites, and rural lands.
tpl.org, 800-714-5263

Union of Concerned Scientists
Coalition of academics clarifying the need for policy change and action.
ucsusa.org, 617-547-5552

Washington Toxics Coalition
Working to eliminate toxic pollution.
watoxics.org, 206-632-1545

Waterkeeper Alliance
Connects and supports local programs to provide a voice for clean waterways.
waterkeeper.org, 914-674-0622

Women's Voices for the Earth
Increasing awareness of the connection between human health and the environment.
womenandenvironment.org, 406-543-3747

Blogs/Internet

apartmenttherapy.com
babble.com
blueegg.com
coopamerica.org/pubs/greenpages
ecofabulous.com

greengirlguide.com
greenopia.com
grist.com
huffingtonpost.com
idealbite.com
inhabitat.com
inspiredprotagonist.com
lime.com
metaefficient.com
sprig.com
sundancechannel.com/thegreen
thecradle.com
thedailygreen.com
thegreenguide.com
thelazyenvironmentalist.com
thesmartmama.com
treehugger.com
triplepundit.com
worldchanging.com
zenhabits.net

Books

Better Basics for the Home by Annie
    Berthold-Bond
Blueprint for a Green School by Jayni
    Chase
The Complete Organic Pregnancy by
    Deirdre Dolan and Alexandra
    Zissu
Cradle to Cradle by William
    McDonough and Michael
    Braungart
The End of Nature by Bill
    McKibben
Food to Live By by Myra Goodman,
    Linda Holland, and Pamela
    McKinstry
The Green Book by Elizabeth Rogers
    and Thomas M. Kostigen

Green Clean by Linda Mason Hunter
    and Mikki Halpin
The Happiest Baby on the Block by
    Harvey Karp
Having Faith by Sandra Steingraber
The Hundred-Year Lie by Randall
    Fitzgerald
The Lorax by Dr. Seuss
Naturally Clean by Jeffrey Hollender,
    Geoff Davis, Meika Hollender,
    and Reed Doyle
The Nature of Design: Ecology,
    Culture, and Human Intention by
    David W. Orr
The Newman's Own Organics Guide to
    a Good Life by Nell Newman and
    Joseph D'Agnese
Ocean Friendly Cuisine by James O.
    Fraioli
Organic Baby: Simple Steps for
    Healthy Living by Kimberly Rider
Parenting from the Inside Out by
    Daniel J. Siegel and Mary Hartzell
The Peaceful Nursery by Laura Forbes
    Carlin and Alison Forbes
The Omnivore's Dilemma by Michael
    Pollan
The Secret History of the War on
    Cancer by Devra Davis
Silent Spring by Rachel Carson
Our Stolen Future by Theo Colborn,
    Dianne Dumanoski, and John
    Peterson Myers
Raising Baby Green by Alan Greene
    with Jeanette Pavini and Theresa
    Foy DiGeronimo
Raising Healthy Children in a Toxic
    World by Philip J. Landrigan,
    Herbert L. Needleman, and Mary
    M. Landrigan

What's Toxic and What's Not by Gary
    Ginsberg and Brian Toal

Magazines

Body + Soul
bodyandsoulmag.com

Cookie
cookiemag.com

Good
goodmagazine.com

Kiwi Magazine
kiwimagonline.com

Mother Jones
motherjones.com

Mothering Magazine
mothering.com

Natural Health Magazine
naturalhealthmag.com

Natural Home and Garden
naturalhomemagazine.com

O at Home
oprah.com

Ode
odemagazine.com

OnEarth
nrdc.org/onearth

Organic Gardening
organicgardening.com

Plenty
plentymag.com

Real Simple
realsimple.com

Utne Reader
utne.com

Vegetarian Times
vegetariantimes.com

Notable Organizations

AirNow
Interactive air quality index site;
check daily air quality.
epa.gov/airnow

**American Public Transportation
Association**
Navigate metropolitan public

transport in your
community.
publictransportation.org,
202-496-4800

**California Office of Environmental
Health Hazard Assessment**
List of art and craft materials that

may not be purchased for use in grades K-6.
oehha.org/education/art/getart.html, 510-622-3200

Center for Environmental Oncology University of Pittsburgh Cancer Institute
Fundamentally synthesizing environmental science data to affect public policy and public education.
environmentaloncology.org, 412-623-3375

Center for a New American Dream
Guide for Americans on responsible consuming.
newdream.org, 877-683-7326

Collaborative for High Performance Schools
Facilitating design of high-performance, environmentally friendly schools.
chps.net/manual/index.htm, 877-642-2477

Computer Take Back Campaign
Protecting the health of electronics users, workers, and communities where electronics are produced and discarded.
computertakeback.com, 512-326-5655

Consumer's Guide to Radon Reduction
For those with elevated radon levels in their home.
radon.com/pubs/consguid.html, 800-767-7236

Co-op America's National Green Pages
Directory of thousands of businesses

that have made commitments to sustainability.
coopamerica.org/pubs/greenpages, 800-584-7336

Cradle to Cradle
Eco-effective design principles and smart product certification process.
mbdc.com, 434-295-1111

Earth Dinner by Organic Valley Farms
Explore about food with your family.
earthdinner.org

Environmental Health Perspectives
Peer-reviewed research and in-depth news on environmental impact on human health.
ehponline.org, 919-653-2581

EPA Children's Environmental Health Hotline
877-590-5437

EPA Healthy School Environments
Providing access to resources to resolve environmental issues in schools.
epa.gov/schools

EPA Indoor Air Quality in Homes
Resource on indoor air quality issues.
epa.gov/iaq/homes, 800-438-4318

EPA Integrated Pest Management (IPM) in Schools
IPM in schools and how to reduce children's exposure to pesticides.
epa.gov/pesticides/ipm, 800-858-7378

EPA Office of Children's Health Protection
Evaluating children's environmental health issues.
epa.gov/children, 202-564-2188

EPA State Water Certification Offices
Organized by state-certified laboratories that test drinking water.
epa.gov/safewater/faq/sco.html, 800-426-4791

EPA Source Water Protection
Protecting drinking water sources from contamination.
epa.gov/safewater/protect.html, 800-426-4791

EPA WaterSense
Promoting home products that conserve water without sacrificing performance.
epa.gov/watersense

Fair Labor Association
Protecting workers' rights and improving working conditions worldwide.
fairlabor.org, 202-898-1000

Fuel Economy
Gas mileage tips, info about energy-efficient vehicles, car comparisons.
fueleconomy.gov, 877-337-3463

GreenHomeGuide
Products and services for homeowners to create greener homes.
greenhomeguide.com

GreenerComputing
Resources for environmentally responsible computing.
greenercomputing.com

GreenDimes
Reduce junk mail by up to 90%, get ten trees planted on your behalf.
greendimes.com

Greenpeace Guide to Greener Electronics
Ranks leading mobile and PC manufacturers on their global and chemical policies.
greenpeace.org

Green Seal
Nonprofit green-certification organization dedicated to protecting the environment.
greenseal.org, 202-872-6400

Household Products Database
Learn about consumer products' potential health effects and safety.
householdproducts.nlm.nih.gov

Janitorial Products Pollution Prevention Project
Fact sheets and tools to evaluate and avoid chemically harsh janitorial products.
wrppn.org/janitorial/jp4.cfm

Mt. Sinai's Center for Children's Health and the Environment
The nation's leading academic research and policy center on environmental health issues.

childenvironment.org,
212-241-7840

National Drinking Water Clearinghouse
Timely drinking water–related information specifically for small communities.
nesc.wvu.edu/ndwc/ndwc_index.htm,
800-624-8301

Oceans Alive
Smart seafood choices, for you and the oceans.
oceansalive.org, 212-505-2100

100 Mile Diet
Local eating for global change.
100milediet.org

Organic Consumers Association
On food safety, industrial agriculture, genetic engineering, and more.
organicconsumers.org, 218-226-4164

Radon Information Center
Resources on radon test kits, links to EPA reports on radon detection and remediation.
radon.com

Safe Drinking Water Hotline
Names of state certification officials.
epa.gov/safewater/hotline,
800-426-4791

Safe Playgrounds Project
Education on minimizing health threats to children from playgrounds;

from the Center for Environmental Health.
safe2play.org, 510-594-9864

SmartWood
Independent auditing, certification, and promotion of FSC-certified forest products.
smartwood.org, 888-693-2784

Sustainable Cotton Project
Raising awareness about harm caused by conventional cotton; enabling safer organic methods.
sustainablecotton.org,
530-756-8518 ext. 34

Sustainable Style Foundation
Information and innovative programs to promote sustainable design.
sustainablestyle.org, 206-324-4850

Sustainable Table
Educating consumers on food-related issues; building community through food.
sustainabletable.org, 212-991-1930

Take the Pledge by Be Truly Green
Info about the health effects of pesticides; alternatives.
refusetousechemlawn.org,
617-292-4821

The Work Group for Community Health and Development
The Community Tool Box offers practical skill building on hundreds of community topics.
ctb.ku.edu, 785-864-0533

ACKNOWLEDGMENTS

This book has truly been a team effort. First, I wish to offer tremendous appreciation and praise to three people who worked tirelessly on the book, with their children (and *their* children) in mind. I could have never done it without you!

Andrew & Alex Postman, and Janelle Sorensen

Special thanks to these individuals who offered guidance and valuable editorial assistance:

Dr. David Carpenter*
Alice I. Chen
James Chuda*
Dr. Theo Colborn*
Dr. Devra Davis*
Mary Martin Gant*
Nancy Greenspan*
Matthew Guma
Tessa Hill*

Erika Imranyi
Dr. Harvey Karp*
Trena Keating
Dr. Philip Landrigan*
Peter Pfeiffer
Carrie Cook Platt*
Jennifer Taggart
Dr. Leonardo Trasande*

Sincere thanks to the following book contributors, longtime friends, community partners, and colleagues, who offered their support for this effort, and who are continually generous with our HCHW work:

John H. Adams
Kelly Austing
Roger Barnett*
Lawrence Bender
Lisa Beres
Davide Berruto
Annie Berthold-Bond
Dr. Kenneth Bock
Jenny Brady
Howard Bragman
Amy Brenneman*
Gerald Breslauer
Lenore Breslauer
Erin Brockovich*
Kevin Brodwick
Natalie Cadranel
Ricky Cappe
Jessica Capshaw
Gigi Lee Chang
Beth Nielsen
   Chapman*
Barry A. Cik
Courteney Cox
Michael Cronan
Sheryl Crow
Blythe Danner
Laura Dern*
Orly Douek
Larry Eason*
Jenna Elfman

Dr. Brenda Eskenazi*
Dr. Ruth Etzel*
Dr. Elaine Faustman*
Jay Feldman*
Helen Ficalora
Rebecca Foster
Shelley Freeman
Marci Frumkin
Tom and Judy
   Gavigan
Betty Ann Gaynor*
Jill Gaynor
Dr. Mitchell Gaynor
Mandy Geisler
Tamar Geller
Anna Getty*
Vanessa Getty
Dr. Gary Ginsberg
Michelle Glenn
Dina Goda
Brooke Golden
Dr. Lynn Goldman*
Myra Goodman*
Dr. Jay Gordon
Jason Graham-Nye
Kim Graham-Nye
Dr. Alan and Cheryl
   Greene*
Doug Greene
Dr. Stanley

Greenspan*
Linda Grey
Tom Hanks
Ben Harper
Maureen Harrington
Chrystie Heimert
Kenneth Heitz
Alice Heller
Joe Henry*
Karin Himba
Jeffrey Hollender*
Kate Hudson
Arianna Huffington
Aisha Ikramuddin
Zem Spire Joaquin*
Jesse Johnson
Rene Jones
Calvin Jung
Melina Kanakaredes
C. J. Kettler*
Gayle King
Jena and Michael
   King*
Michelle Kleinert
Danica Krislovich
Cindra and Alan
   Ladd, Jr.
Margaret Leidy
Norman and Lyn
   Lear

Michelle Kydd Lee
Luanna Lindsey*
Russell Long
Linda Loudermilk
Craig H. Lyons
Kristie Macosko
Tobey Maguire
Josie Maran
Ashlee Margolis
Frank Marshall
Tasneem Matola
William
  McDonough*
Stephan McGuire
Nicole Meadow
Jen Meyer
Kelly Chapman
  Meyer
Al Meyerhoff
Nina Montée*
Sara
  Bramin-Mooser
Carolyn Murphy
Tanya and David
  Murphy*
Dr. Herbert L.
  Needleman
Nell Newman
Olivia Newton-John*

Michelle Obama
Robyn O'Brien
Tim O'Shea
Dr. David Orr
Gwyneth Paltrow
Raina Penchansky
Holly Robinson Peete
Dr. John Peters*
Warren Porter
Akasha Richmond
Anne Robertson*
Dr. Leslie Robison*
Laurie Rocke
Elizabeth Rogers
Cheryl Roth
Keri Russell
Kelly Rutherford
Charles Schmidt
Rachel Sarnoff
Sandra Schubert
Dr. Joel Schwartz*
Laura Turner Seydel
Brooke Shields
Tim Smith
Bahar Soomekh
Andy Spahn
Kate Capshaw
  Spielberg
Steven Spielberg

Dr. Sandra
  Steingraber*
Meryl Streep*
Duke Stump
Chip Sullivan
Talley Summerlin
Elizabeth Sword
Paige Goldberg
  Tolmach
Ron Vigdor
Amanda Walker
Leah Walton
Dr. John Wargo*
Dr. Jeffrey
  Werber
Sheldon
  Whitehouse
Elizabeth Wiatt
Jan Williams
Sarah Williams
Vanessa Williams
Cyd Wilson
Rita Wilson
Kori E.
  Wilson-Griffin
Suzanne and Bob
  Wright*
Noah Wyle

*Board of Directors, Board of Advisors, or Scientific Advisory Committee

PERMISSIONS

Grateful acknowledgment is made for permission to reprint the recipes and information on the following pages:

Pages 23 and 44: Reprinted from *Home Enlightenment* by Annie B. Bond. Copyright © 2005 by Annie B. Bond. Permission granted by Rodale, Inc., Emmaus, PA 18098. Available wherever books are sold or directly from the publisher by calling (800) 848-4735, or visit their Web site at www.rodalestore.com.

Pages 110, 164, and 225: Reprinted from *What's Toxic, What's Not* by Gary Ginsberg and Brian Toal, M.S.P.H. Copyright © 2006 by Gary Ginsberg and Brian Toal. Used by permission of Berkley Publishing Group, a division of Penguin Group (USA) Inc.

ABOUT HEALTHY CHILD
HEALTHY WORLD

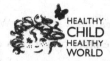

A national 501(c)3 nonprofit organization, Healthy Child Healthy World is dedicated to protecting children's health and well-being from harmful environmental exposures. Through education and prevention strategies, Healthy Child informs parents, supports protective policies, and engages communities to make responsible choices to create healthy environments for children and families.

Healthy Child Healthy World was founded by James and Nancy Chuda in 1991 after their daughter Colette died from Wilms' tumor, a rare form of nonhereditary cancer. The organization is governed by a volunteer board of directors and a distinguished board of advisors and scientific committee, and is strengthened by community and business partners.

Join our effort in one of the most important public health and environmental movements of our time. See healthychild.org for more information.

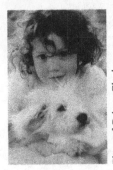

Photo of Colette Chuda
by Irene Newton-John

Colette's Inspiration

Every day of our daughter's life was a gift. We weren't young parents, and her arrival marked the start of a joyous chapter that fulfilled our yearnings for a family. Then, at age four, Colette was diagnosed with Wilms' tumor, a rare form of cancer.

After a yearlong struggle, we lost the love and light of our lives. Colette was five.

As parents, we believed intuitively that something in the environment triggered our daughter's cancer. In our journey to uncover what made our Colette sick, we recognized that more research on environmental exposures and toxic substances in everyday products was necessary, and that more appropriate protection standards, both legislative and corporate, should be established to prioritize children's and family health.

We turned our pain into a passion and founded the nonprofit organization Healthy Child Healthy World (formerly CHEC) with the help of family and friends, including our best friend, Olivia Newton-John, to serve as an educational platform for children's environmental health, one that embraced credible information with positive strategies.

We understand only too well that a parent's single greatest wish is for his or her child to be healthy. We hope this book, and this organization inspired by Colette, will share the many insights and practical solutions that can help you to take greater charge of your children's health.

—Nancy and James Chuda, cofounders,
Healthy Child Healthy World

CONTRIBUTORS

Amy Brenneman

Erin Brockovich

Jessica Capshaw

Gigi Lee Chang

Dr. Theo Colborn

Courteney Cox

Sheryl Crow

Dr. Devra Davis

Laura Dern

Jenna Elfman

Tamar Geller

Anna Getty

Dr. Gary Ginsberg

Myra Goodman

Jason and Kim Graham-Nye

Dr. Alan Greene

Tom Hanks

Tessa Hill

Jeffrey Hollender

Kate Hudson

Zem Spire Joaquin

Melina Kanakaredes

Dr. Harvey Karp

Gayle King

Dr. Philip Landrigan

Russell Long

Tobey Maguire

Josie Maran

William McDonough

Nicole Meadow

Jen Meyer

Carolyn Murphy

Tanya Murphy

Nell Newman

Michelle Obama

Robyn O'Brien

Dr. David Orr

Holly Robinson Peete

Gwyneth Paltrow

Peter Pfeiffer

Keri Russell

Laura Turner Seydel

Brooke Shields

Dr. Sandra Steingraber

Meryl Streep

Jennifer Taggart

Paige Goldberg Tolmach

Vanessa Williams

Rita Wilson

Noah Wyle

INDEX